PRAISE FOR

Aging with

GRACE

"Part of a body of new research showing that a life well lived . . . may protect against . . . life-threatening illness."—*US News and World Report*

"A wonderfully warm and illuminating account . . . a rare book for the way it combines cutting-edge science with an inside view of how that knowledge is being created."—*The Guardian* (UK)

"The Nun Study represents an absolutely unique American treasure and resource for all of us. The gems that Dr. Snowdon and his colleagues have unearthed will not only change the way you look at yourself and the aging people around you, they'll serve as catalysts for aging research for many years to come."
　　　—Ronald Petersen, Ph.D., M.D., director of the Alzheimer's Disease
　　　　Research Center, Mayo Clinic

"There are lessons for all of us in this moving account of the School Sisters of Notre Dame and their commitment to help us find the causes of Alzheimer's disease. I came away with a new respect for the power of faith as well as the beauty and complexity of the human brain."
　　　—Virginia M. Bell, M.S.W., co-author of *The Best Friends Approach to*
　　　　Alzheimer's Care

"David Snowdon leads us through the enthralling scientific, but also very personal, journey that he has been taking with the School Sisters of Notre Dame. The revelations along the way show us there is so much we can all do to alter for the better how we age, and ultimately how long we live. It is a journey not to be missed!"
　—Thomas Perls, M.D., M.P.H., Professor of Medicine, Harvard Medical School

"A beautiful story. Families will find hope and support through the commitment of the sisters who have dedicated their lives to helping others enjoy the gift of life as long as possible."
　　—Sigmund Tomkalski, Executive Director, Southeastern Wisconsin Chapter,
　　　Alzheimer Association

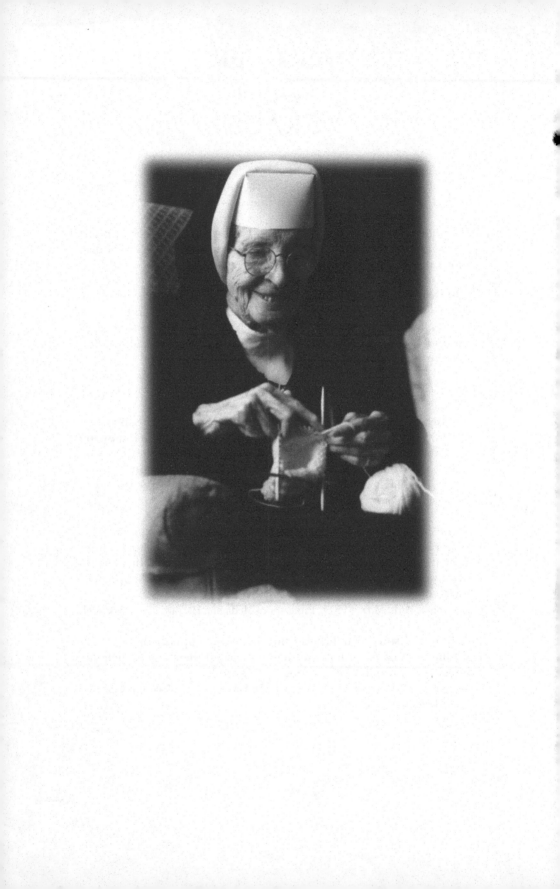

Aging with
GRACE

What the Nun Study
Teaches Us About
Leading Longer, Healthier,
and
More Meaningful Lives

DAVID SNOWDON, PH.D.

Bantam Books
New York Toronto London Sydney Auckland

This edition contains the complete text
of the original hardcover edition.
NOT ONE WORD HAS BEEN OMITTED.

AGING WITH GRACE
A Bantam Book

PUBLISHING HISTORY
Bantam hardcover edition published / May 2001
Bantam trade paperback edition / May 2002

Book design by O'Lanso Gabbidon

Front cover photo © Lee P. Thomas: Nun Study participant
Sister Andrea Carron, a School Sister of Notre Dame from St. Louis

Cover design by Aenee Sheen

Library of Congress Catalog Card Number: 00-069658
For information address: Bantam Books.

ISBN 978-0-553-38092-7

Published simultaneously in the United States and Canada

Bantam Books are published by Bantam Books, a division of Random House, Inc.
Its trademark, consisting of the words "Bantam Books" and the portrayal of a
rooster, is Registered in U.S. Patent and Trademark Office and in other countries.
Marca Registrada. Bantam Books, New York, New York.

PRINTED IN THE UNITED STATES OF AMERICA

In gratitude for the participation and prayers
of the thousands of dedicated School Sisters of Notre Dame
in the seven provinces in the United States

Baltimore, Maryland
Chicago, Illinois
Dallas, Texas
Mankato, Minnesota
Milwaukee, Wisconsin
St. Louis, Missouri
Wilton, Connecticut

And for my parents

Hank and Barbara Snowdon

Contents

A Note on Privacy

——— ❦ ———

The School Sisters of Notre Dame who participate in the Nun Study have opened their lives and personal histories to us in an extraordinary way, trusting that we will use this information wisely in our quest to understand Alzheimer's disease. I am deeply grateful to them, and also deeply aware of my responsibility to protect their privacy. In this book a sister is identified by her real name (including her family name) only when she has given us permission to do so. For a number of reasons, other sisters are identified by a first name or religious name only. These names have all been changed, and other identifying characteristics of these sisters' lives have been changed as well. The scientific details, however, remain accurate for all sisters in the study.

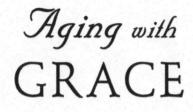

Aging with GRACE

Prologue

Other Worlds

I recall a bright Saturday afternoon on a highway outside Redlands, California, my hometown. I'm five years old. My mother pilots our light green Ford Ranch wagon south toward San Diego. She is secretary to our parish priest, Father Henry Keane, and on this day she is chauffeuring five nuns who teach at Sacred Heart, the school where I will enroll the following year.

It's 1957, and none of the sisters has a driver's license, much less a car. Two sisters sit up front with my mother and three sit in the backseat, lined up like fence posts in their full black-and-white wool serge habits. That leaves me, the little boy with the butch haircut, crammed into the rear luggage compartment, the space usually reserved for our fox terrier, Spot. Broiling heat from the Santa Ana winds cooks the car's interior, but the five overdressed sisters remain stoic, their pale faces framed by the perfect ovals of their white wimples. Keeping vigil over all of us is St. Christopher, a small, cream-colored statue anchored to the dashboard.

From my perch in the back, I peer out at the people in passing cars. Most of them are tanned and clothed in the diverse colors of southern California. They turn with startled expressions to stare into our old green boat, packed to the gunnels with nuns. It is then that I realize that these brides of Christ, who have taken vows of poverty, chastity, and obedience, are as mysterious to most outsiders as they are to me. It is as though they were inhabitants of a different world.

—

Nearly four decades later, investigating that world would become my life's work. From the boy who dreamed of being a gymnast and a farmer, I have morphed into a medical detective, an epidemiologist looking for clues to the mysteries of aging. Now I want to know what secrets I can learn from these religious women about one of the most puzzling other worlds that science has ever probed: Alzheimer's disease.

Religious groups, with their carefully regulated lives and copious records, are ideal subjects for epidemiologists. Why, the Nun Study asks, do some of the sisters age gracefully, continuing to teach and serve, retaining their mental faculties into their eighties and nineties, even past one hundred? Why do others—who have lived such similar lives—appear to lose themselves, forgetting their closest friends and relatives and, in the end, becoming almost wholly disconnected from the world around them?

For nearly fifteen years now, the Nun Study has led me deeper and deeper into the world of aging and Alzheimer's, the questions becoming ever more layered and intriguing, the possible answers more meaningful to all of us. What my coworkers and I have learned so far has challenged some of the basic scientific tenets about Alzheimer's disease, which afflicts up to 45 percent of Americans over eighty-five years of age. Aging may be inevitable, but as our research shows, Alzheimer's disease may not be—and we have uncovered promising clues about how to avoid it.

Along the way I have developed a strong attachment to the School Sisters of Notre Dame, a remarkable group of women—678 of whom have selflessly given themselves to this project. Many of the sisters at the seven main Notre Dame convents in the United States have become part of my extended family, and my visits more closely resemble a drop-in from a nephew—or, more precisely, a great-nephew—than those of a detached, objective scientist venturing into the field to collect data. Which means that on each visit to a convent, I risk discovering that I am losing a friend.

—

I met Sister Maria in 1991 at Elm Grove, a convent built over a century ago in a suburb of Milwaukee, Wisconsin. She was then seventy-eight years old and recently retired from her work as a seamstress for the community. I was immediately drawn to her. Sister Maria was not a "modern" nun—she wore the traditional full habit every day—but she had a wry sense of humor and a wonderful, ready smile. And there was something special about being in her presence. As her nephew—himself a priest—once said, "Maria already lived partly in heaven."

Sister Maria also took a liking to me, and whenever I came to stay at the convent, she would look after me—asking about my life, telling me about her childhood in Germany, making sure I knew the meal and Mass schedule, and stocking the refrigerator in my convent room with beer.

Maria was among the first group of Milwaukee sisters to join the Nun Study. She took her initial mental examination when she was seventy-nine years old. This hourlong battery of tests assesses memory, concentration, language, visual-spatial abilities, and orientation to time and place. The tests remain the same from year to year, because we want to capture the unique "fingerprint," or pattern of change, in each woman.

Another sister, a member of our research team, administered the Delayed Word Recall test, the most sensitive indicator of forgetfulness. Sister Marlene Manney, the examiner, showed Sister Maria ten index cards, each with a different word printed on it, and asked Maria to say each word as she flipped the cards.

This was done three times. The words were:*

Leg
Cheese
Tent
Motor
Flower
Stamp
Cup
King
Forest
Menu

After this "learning phase," Sister Marlene ran Sister Maria through other tests for five minutes to distract her. She then asked Sister Maria to recall as many of the ten words as she could. Her response was recorded on videotape.

"A few minutes ago I asked you to learn a list of ten words, which you read one at a time from cards," Sister Marlene said. "Now I want you to recall as many of those ten words as you can."

---

*To maintain the integrity of the test, I have substituted different but similar words.

"Most are gone with the wind," Sister Maria replied softly, swatting the air with both hands, as if dismissing the possibility that she could do it. Her voice still carried the German accent of her childhood.

"*Leg.*" She paused for five seconds.

"*King.*" Twenty seconds of silence passed.

"*Motor.*" After another long pause, in which she turned her head back and forth to search her memory, she finally said, "*Stamp.*"

Sister Maria's recall of only four of the ten words barely met the criteria for normal short-term memory.

One year later, when she was eighty, Sister Maria took a second, identical exam.

"Tell me as many of those ten words as you can remember."

"I don't think I remember that. . . ." Sister Maria's sentence trailed off as she gravely looked at the examiner.

"You read them when I flipped the cards. You read them over three times."

"Did I?"

"Can you remember any of those, Sister?" Sister Marlene was gentle in her prompts.

Sister Maria's smile came through even on the grainy videotape. "I don't think so. . . . *Leg.*"

"That's right, Sister, those are the ones."

"*Stamp,*" Sister Maria said, studying the ceiling in search of the other words. "What else? What else?" she said to herself, shaking her head. "They're gone."

Now Sister Maria's response was typical of someone in the early stages of Alzheimer's disease.

When she was eighty-two years old, Sister Maria took the exam for the last time. By then she had moved from the Elm Grove convent to nearby Marian Catholic, a nursing home.

"Tell me as many of those ten words as you can remember."

"I cannot use these?" She pointed to the stack of index

cards in front of her that held the words. "Then I could do it!" Sister Maria and Sister Marlene both laughed.

Becoming more serious, Sister Maria folded her hands in front of her, tapping the table with her fingers, and repeated, "Ten words." Again the frustration on her face set in as she searched her memory.

"Leg." Sister Maria shook her head. "Isn't that something? I thought it's done, and then I forget it."

She waved her hand over the stack of cards like a magician and smiled. Had any of the other sisters remembered all ten words? she asked. When Sister Marlene told her that some of them had, Sister Maria seemed puzzled. Her smile disappeared.

"Many things in life are not worth remembering," she said, staring down at her hands. "Now I wish I could remember."

That day Sister Maria also took a standard test called the Mini-Mental State Exam.

"What is the year?"

"Nineteen hundred and . . . and . . . I can't even think of the year. Isn't that something? I should be able to say that in my sleep."

"That's all right. What is the season of the year?"

"It's going to be . . . I can't say."

"What month is it?" Sister Marlene recorded in her notes that it was May.

"March? I feel ashamed that I don't remember that."

"That's all right, Sister. You're doing okay. Without looking at your watch or a clock, about what time is it now?"

"It's morning."

"What time is it?"

"It's very early in the morning. Maybe around eight o'clock." Sister Marlene recorded in her notes that it was actually 2:28 P.M.

"What state are we in?"

Sister Maria paused. "Isn't that something? I don't know."

"What city or town are we in?"

"Mequon? Are we in Mequon? I don't know." Sister Maria had lived in a convent in Mequon, a town in Wisconsin, for many years earlier in her life. For the past twelve years, however, she had lived in Milwaukee. Later in the test, when Sister Marlene asked her to compose a sentence, she wrote, "I love to be here." But where was *here?*

—

I visited Sister Maria at the Marian Catholic Nursing Home in March 1995, shortly after her last exam. Walking down the sixth-floor hallway, I passed a few of the aged residents sitting in their wheelchairs staring blankly into space. Most of them were laypeople who shared the same floor as the sisters. One of them, a man who looked to be in his eighties, called out to me in Polish, as if asking for help. I smiled and touched his shoulder as I walked by.

When I reached Sister Maria's room, I found her lying on her bed, still as a corpse, fully clothed in her black-and-white habit, with her hands placed symmetrically on her stomach. Her fingers clutched sky-blue rosary beads, and her eyes were closed under her thick glasses. If I had not known better, I would have thought she had gone to meet her Lord. But Sister Maria had developed a habit of "playing dead" and praying to God to retrieve her from this world.

Sister Maria had become alarmingly frail since I'd seen her last. Lying there on the bed, she looked so peaceful that I hesitated to wake her. But I was leaving Milwaukee in a few hours, and I knew it would be at least six months before I returned.

My hands applied the lightest pressure on her fragile shoulders.

"Sister Maria," I whispered. "It's Dr. Snowdon, Sister. I'm leaving soon, and I just want to say goodbye."

Her eyes opened. She greeted me with her familiar smile, nodding silently.

As a boy, I grew up somewhat shy and uncomfortable around others. Yet around Sister Maria, I'd always felt at ease with myself and the world. I could sit with her for long periods without saying a word, completely comfortable in the silence. Now I wanted to tell her how grateful I was for her friendship and how much I had learned from her, but I did not want to embarrass her. I thought for a minute and decided to let her in on a secret.

"You know, Sister Maria," I said, "I really like you. You're one of my favorite sisters."

Sister Maria adjusted her eyeglasses and slowly sat up, her rosary rocking back and forth in her hand like a metronome, marking the moments it took to right herself. Finally she smiled at me again, her face glowing.

"I love you, too," she said softly.

She then shifted uncomfortably and leaned toward me to examine my face. Her eyes narrowed into thin creases; her eyebrows bunched together as if my face were a puzzle she could not solve.

"Who are you?"

You are never prepared for the devastation Alzheimer's brings. I wanted to say something—I needed to say something—but I was afraid that anything I said would make things worse. I took her hand and squeezed it gently. She looked down at my hand, and her question seemed to slip away as easily as it had come. Slowly she looked up at me with another serene smile.

It was all I could do to smile back.

———

"I hope I die before I get old," sang The Who in "My Generation." I am part of the very generation they were singing to, and many of us who grew up with that anthem have learned, as we ourselves have aged, how naive a conceit that is. The School Sisters of Notre Dame have shown me that old age is not something to fear and revile. It can be a time of promise and renewal, of watching with a knowing eye, of accepting the lessons that life has taught and, if possible, passing them on to the generations that will follow. What I have learned from the sisters—many of whom remain mentally robust after a century of life—is that The Who had it exactly backward. I hope I get old before I die.

Yet I also hope that on the day before I leave this earth, I will still have a mind that can communicate with my limbs, allow me to feel elation or regret, and properly process a sunrise's brilliance, a freshly mowed lawn's aroma, the chill of a fall night, and the love of family and friends. I want to feel that I have completed my mission in life, that I have made some small difference in this world. And I want to remember all that I can for as long as I can.

Near the end of her life, Sister Maria confided to me her greatest fear. "I am ready to go," she said, "I want to go. I have waited all my life for this. But now I worry God has forgotten me." God did not forget Sister Maria. She died peacefully nine months after our last visit, and for that I am relieved. What makes me angry and sad is that Alzheimer's disease robbed her of so many of the pleasures and rewards of growing old.

What makes me hopeful, however, is that we are learning from studying Maria and hundreds of other sisters how to achieve the promise of old age—or, as our Nun Study motto expresses it: "That You May Have Life to the Full."

1

――――― ● ―――――

The Road to Good Counsel Hill

They will open up to you, but only if you give of yourself first.
—Sister Carmen Burg

On a spring morning in 1986, when the midwestern snowpack finally had begun to melt and the change of seasons encouraged new ideas to sprout, I sat nervously in the reception room of a convent in St. Paul, Minnesota, with a new idea of my own. I had come here to meet Sister Carmen Burg, who would either help my idea take root or wish me luck and send me on my way. I feared that she had bad news for me.

As an assistant professor of epidemiology at the University of Minnesota, I was struggling mightily to find my niche. In the competitive world of scientific research, especially at a large institution, I knew I had little time to establish my value to the department. All too frequently I remembered my chairman's words: "It's nice to be independent, but *you must be funded.*"

Sister Carmen was an elected leader of one of Minnesota's largest groups of Catholic nuns, the School Sisters of Notre Dame. Nearly two hundred sisters lived at the Good Counsel Hill convent in Mankato, ninety miles southwest of St. Paul. I had contacted Sister Carmen to propose a research project involving the nuns. Now I worried that she had offered to meet me here—before I ever got to Mankato—so that it would be less awkward to turn me down. Underscoring my anxiety were images that had been seared into my memory at Sacred Heart elementary school. Most of the sisters had been serious, take-no-prisoners disciplinarians.

I had learned what I knew about the School Sisters of Notre Dame from Nora Keenan, a graduate student in our department. Nora had an unusual background for an epidemiologist: She had previously been one of the Notre Dames and had lived at the Mankato convent. She explained to me that her former congregation had originated in Bavaria in 1833, at a time of great political and social upheaval. The founder was a teacher at a parochial school, Caroline Gerhardinger, who later took the religious name Mary Teresa of Jesus. Mother Teresa, as she was known, believed that society could be transformed through the family, and that her call was to provide education and spiritual formation for girls— particularly poor girls in rural areas. Shortly after the congregation was established, millions of Germans—driven by crop failure and revolution—began to emigrate to the United States, and the American bishops asked Mother Teresa to consider a new frontier for her mission. Together with four other sisters, she arrived at a forest settlement in Pennsylvania in 1847. From there, the congregation had moved west and south with the immigrants, founding schools and convents throughout North America. By 1986, the congregation (now based in Rome) had more than seven thousand sisters in nearly thirty countries. The Mankato convent—one of seven provincial motherhouses in this country—had been established in 1912.

Nora's account immediately sparked my interest. As I told her one day over lunch, I had built my career so far around studying unique populations of religious groups. For my Ph.D. thesis at Minnesota, I had joined an ongoing study of the Lutheran Brotherhood and investigated whether cancer and heart disease had any links to alcohol use. I then worked at California's Loma Linda Medical College, investigating the impact of diet on the health of Seventh-day Adventists. Now that I was back at Minnesota, I wanted to study aging and health, and I suspected that nuns or priests—I did not really have a preference—would offer unique clues. It was then that Nora had offered an introduction to Sister Carmen.

My nervous wait ended when a short, smiling woman came into the reception room and held out her hand. Sister Carmen was dressed in a simple white blouse, camel-colored cardigan, and long plaid skirt. Only a small pin over her heart signaled her membership in the School Sisters of Notre Dame. I had forgotten that since my days at Sacred Heart school, the reforms of the Second Vatican Council (or Vatican II) had made the black-and-white habit an option. Now in her early sixties, Sister Carmen wore large glasses, and behind them I could see the intelligent, patient eyes of a woman who had taught thousands of children. After we had chatted for a few minutes, she got right to the point.

"You know, Dr. Snowdon," she said in her distinct midwestern accent, "I love being a nun. Sisters are as human as the next person. But my question is, why on earth do you want to study nuns?"

She listened attentively as I described my past work with Lutherans and Adventists. I explained to Sister Carmen that these religious groups kept extensive membership lists and historical records that made them ideal subjects for epidemiological studies. And the members often had similar lifestyles, which enabled researchers to make powerful comparisons of factors connected to illness or health. Nuns had even more similar histories. They do not smoke. They are celibate. They have similar jobs and income, and they receive similar health care for most of their lives. All of these factors reduce the confounding variables—such as poverty and lack of health care—that can cloud the meaning of data. Outside a laboratory, it would be hard to find as pure an environment for research.

In fact, I went on, nuns had already played a crucial role in expanding our understanding of two devastating diseases that afflict women: breast cancer and cervical cancer. In the 1950s scientists observed that nuns had an unusually high risk for breast cancer. This led researchers to examine overall breast cancer rates more closely, comparing single to married women. It emerged that single women, like nuns, also had a high risk of breast cancer. The variable turned out to be pregnancy and the hormonal changes it causes. Much of today's understanding of how hormones affect breast health had its origin in this research.

Several famous studies, on the other hand, have reported cervical cancer to be rare in nuns and common in prostitutes, I offered, immediately realizing how odd this must have sounded to Sister Carmen. In this case, it was a sexually transmitted virus that ultimately emerged as the link to cancer. "Again, it isn't difficult to make the connection," I added.

"No, it isn't," she agreed.

I gladly changed the subject to aging and the purpose of my visit. "I'm hoping the study of the School Sisters of Notre Dame will lead to some major clues about aging and disease," I said. "Ultimately, I want to increase our knowledge and help people live longer, better lives."

Sister Carmen brightened when she heard this. If she was

bothered by the vagueness—or vastness—of what I was proposing, she didn't let on. She sat quietly for a minute.

"Let me tell you, Dr. Snowdon," she began. "We have always believed in the power of knowledge and ideas. A large part of our mission has *always* been teaching. Over ninety percent of our sisters have been teachers at one time. Some of our older sisters taught in towns that had no schools before they arrived.

"Our sisters have spent their entire adult lives trying to help other people in the community. Even in their retirement, they have a deep passion and drive to help others. I think they would see your study as a way to continue their lifelong mission of helping others, of educating others."

"Yes, I hope so," I said.

Sister Carmen paused again and then let out a big, contented sigh. "Okay," she said, as only a Minnesotan can.

"Okay?" I was confused. "You mean—"

"Wait." She raised her open hand and stopped me in mid-sentence. "I'll move forward with your request, but you need to listen carefully to what I am about to say. No matter what you do, I want you to remember who these women are. They are real people. Very dear to us. They are holy people, too. I don't want you to treat them as research subjects. Get to know them. Understand that many of the older sisters were the teachers or mentors of the younger sisters, and we treat them with the care and respect they deserve. We will expect nothing less from you."

I was a little stunned by Sister Carmen's statement. My prior research projects had included tens of thousands of participants, and I knew them only through their medical records and the questionnaires they had filled out. All researchers are taught that scientific objectivity depends on keeping one's distance from the people one studies. I had no idea how I could fulfill her request, so I simply nodded and said, "I'll do my best."

Sister Carmen gave me this parting advice: "They will open up to you," she said, "but only if you give of yourself first."

——

If Sister Carmen had asked me how I became an epidemiologist, I would have had to answer, "Chickens."

Puberty took away my lithe frame, ruining my imagined future as a gymnast, so I needed something new to do after school. Unlike my two older brothers, I had little interest in football or baseball. Being a teen also meant that I badly wanted to be different from my brothers—and everyone else. So I decided to take up a hobby my father had pursued when he was a child: raising chickens and selling their eggs. With his help, I built a couple of coops in our suburban backyard and bought some multicolored bantam chickens at a local farm.

Bantams are the most petite breed of poultry, and they only occasionally lay eggs, which also are quite small. When I realized that these miniature chickens would produce only miniature profits, I began to do my homework. I became a student of chickens.

I read every book in the library about chickens, requested every pamphlet on chicken farming available from the United States Department of Agriculture, and wrote every hatchery in the state asking for information on their chicks. I finally decided to breed Rhode Island Reds, which my father had raised, both because they had excellent egg production and because they had enough meat on their bones to make a decent meal. I bought a trio of Reds, two hens and a rooster, from a noted breeder in Illinois, who shipped them by train to my home in California.

My chicken hobby became my passion. Business began to boom, and I made more money on my egg route than my friends made on their newspaper routes. I became "David the

Eggman," a nickname that riffed off Beatles lyrics and made me proud.

My flock grew to nearly a hundred Rhode Island Reds, and I monitored my population closely. I weighed each bird weekly and charted individual egg production. I vaccinated every chick. Any bird that fell ill went into isolation so as not to infect others. I installed the best watering system I could afford, fed them high-quality feed, kept refining their housing conditions, and when necessary treated them with antibiotics. It was pure economics: The longer I could keep each bird alive, well, and productive, the more money I could make. I began systematically studying ways to maintain my flock's health and well-being, which led to several blue-ribbon birds that I showed at the San Bernardino County Fair.

Although I did not know it at the time, my chickens taught me the fundamentals of epidemiology. Understanding the causes of a disease in a population can lead to prevention strategies—and it's far more effective to prevent disease than to treat it after it has occurred. To study the factors that cause disease, we need to compare individuals in a population, from the direly ill to the remarkably healthy as well as the ones in between. Disease is a process, and the conditions of early life—whether chosen or imposed—often cause or prevent later problems.

Finally, my flock also introduced me to a central focus of gerontology: the importance of maintaining function and of understanding the key points along a continuum, from highly productive to completely disabled. For my chickens, the question was pretty simple: How often and long would they continue to lay eggs? Successful aging in a human being is more complicated, as maintaining both physical and mental function requires an intricate interplay of myriad factors. Nonetheless, the basic principles are similar to those I learned in my own backyard.

I've always enjoyed the two-hour drive down U.S. 169 from the Twin Cities to Mankato. I made the trip for the first time two weeks after my meeting with Sister Carmen Burg. The road keeps company with the Minnesota River much of the way and runs through rolling fields of soybeans and corn. Elm trees shade the white farmhouses, and silos sit next to red barns—the kind of comfortable midwestern landscape that might appear in a child's picture book. It was a six-day trek in 1852, the year Mankato was named with the Sioux word for "blue earth." The bluish-tinted clay soil is still visible along the roadside as you approach the town. The French explorer Pierre LeSueur was so sure it contained copper that he shipped two tons of the stuff back to France in 1701—only to be given the disappointing news that it was worthless.

Good Counsel Hill—or the Hill, as it is known in these parts—is in the northern section of town. As the road winds upward past the high school track and soccer field, the spire of the convent's chapel jumps into view. The aqua-colored water tower confirms that you are in the right place: Good Counsel, it says in bold block letters.

Past a garden planted with azaleas, roses, and wildflowers, the convent's main entrance is guarded by two marble angels. I still miss the presence of Sister Timona, who was the unofficial night sentry during my early visits. Sister Timona maintained her post in full black-and-white habit, resting from time to time in one of the wheelchairs kept by the door. This was her only concession to her eighty-nine years of age. She would call out cheerfully to the nurses at shift change, and she soon greeted me just as warmly.

The convent is made up of four no-frills red brick buildings, and the hallways can sometimes feel like a maze. But the feeling of orderliness and calm is palpable the minute you enter.

To the left of the main entrance is the community room, lit by high windows and furnished with comfortable sofas and rockers. Brass lamps and green plants sit on the side tables, along with copies of *Catholic Digest* and *Time* and glass jars of peppermints.

There's a large dining table at one end of the room, and next to it is a smaller table where a few sisters—the "night owls"—sometimes play cards late in the evening, which means eight-thirty or nine, except for Fridays, when the sisters stay up a little later for popcorn and pop. The sisters are big on games. Competition is stiff on everything from dominoes to Triple Yahtzee, bridge to Scrabble, Boggle to cribbage, and a dice game called Fill or Bust. I learned quickly that I'd have to pay full attention if I wanted to keep up with the play—and the scoring.

For my first visit, I had planned a short presentation about the study I hoped to do. Sister Rita Schwalbe, one of the administrators at the convent, introduced me to the hundred or so sisters who had come to hear me. "He's here to observe us, and he's going to be here a lot," Sister Rita said.

My aim at first was modest and protean: I wanted to investigate aging, though I still had only sketchy ideas about what it was I hoped to learn. Some of the sisters had a fire in their eyes as they listened to me, absorbing every word. Others fell asleep in their wheelchairs. I felt off balance, still touched by my grade-school fear of nuns.

After I spoke, many of the sisters gathered around, waiting patiently for their turn to welcome me to their home. "I was a college professor for forty-eight years and I missed only two days of classes!" one of them said proudly. "I'm seventy-five years old and I feel great," proclaimed another.

I was astounded to learn that one sister had taken the bus from Red Wing, a hundred miles away, to attend. I was even more astounded when she told me she was seventy-nine and still working as the official parish visitor for St. Joseph's Church; she walked everywhere in that hilly town, calling on the elderly and sick and delivering the Holy Eucharist to the homebound. She peppered me with questions about my work, and I took careful note of her name: Sister Nicolette Welter. Here was a sister who surely had much to teach me about successful aging. Her body had not failed her, and her mind was keenly alive to new ideas and possibilities.

I knew that I would have to narrow down my thinking to come up with a manageable research topic, and I began making regular trips to Mankato, hoping to find a focus. I also wanted to honor my promise to Sister Carmen and get to know the sisters. My own grandparents had died when I was quite young, and like many members of my generation, I had grown up without any significant contact with old people. I simply did not know what to expect.

I stationed myself in the community room, guessing that its central location and proximity to the chapel would make it easier for the sisters to approach me. My guest room was right across the hall, next to an alcove housing a statue of Mother Caroline Friess, the first leader of the School Sisters of Notre Dame in America. Mother Caroline, I quickly learned, had arrived from Bavaria with Mother Teresa in 1847 and spent the next five decades establishing more than two hundred schools.

The sisters passed by my station every day on their way to the chapel—for lauds (morning prayer) at 7:45, Mass at 11:00, and vespers at 4:00. Next to the chapel doors was a bulletin board covered with small notices, or "intentions":

Mr. Joseph Berkley of St. Peter is having surgery Thursday, please pray for him and his family.

Pray for our sisters in Central America, who are trying to help the earthquake victims.

Mrs. Dee Morris recently passed away, leaving behind two young children and a loving husband. Please pray for her and her family.

At prayers and Mass the chapel filled with sisters, some fully mobile, others with walkers, and many in wheelchairs. The front section was reserved for "those with wheels." Some sisters read from large-print missals; others used magnifying glasses to see the print. The hard-of-hearing had headphones to help them follow the service.

I was shy by nature, and in many cases it was the sisters who made the first move. One of the first to befriend me was Sister Clarissa Gores, whose biological sisters Liguori and Amalia were also School Sisters of Notre Dame. I would meet her breezing down the hallway in the motorized cart she called her "Chevy," or join her to watch Minnesota Twins games on television with Sister Amalia and a few other sports fans. They knew all the players and could outtalk me on baseball lore any day of the week.

I was surprised to discover that there were many other "sister sisters" among the nuns. The "Gores girls," as they were called, had been separated at a very young age after their mother died, and they especially enjoyed their retirement together. Sister Liguori had moved to the assisted-living wing of the convent, and Sister Clarissa rode over in her Chevy to visit three or four times a day.

At mealtimes, Sister Borgia Leuther often invited me to sit next to her. Sister Borgia was born in 1895 and had taught for fifty years. Now, in her retirement, she created handmade greeting cards by pasting bits of ribbon and dried flowers to white card stock. My mother loved Sister Borgia's cards, which I would buy for her at the convent's gift shop.

Later, as we became better acquainted, Sister Borgia invited me to her room to show me her latest designs. The room was sparse and tile-floored, with only a bed, dresser, small desk and chair, and one upholstered chair for visitors. But Sister Borgia had covered every surface with religious pictures, family photos, books, and memorabilia. It was something like an unusually clean college dorm room—complete with the bathroom down the hall.

As I grew familiar with the convent routine, I felt at times like a botanist who wanders into a tropical rainforest and sees thousands of beautiful flowers worthy of study but cannot decide where to start. I would meet one octogenarian sister who was translating German into English, another who was writing a letter to her congressperson, and a third who was typing her memoirs in the library, and I would want to study whether mental activity warded off memory loss. Or I would walk by the physical therapy room and see seven or eight elderly sisters hard at work, one on the treadmill, two others hoisting three-pound arm weights, another pedaling an exercise bike with a towel draped over her knees for modesty. Perhaps, I would think, I should investigate the effects of exercise on longevity. Or I would sit down to a hearty noon meal of chicken noodle soup, sloppy joe, green bean casserole, and German chocolate cake and wonder if I should continue the kind of dietary study that had launched my career as an epidemiologist.

I was also struck by the stark contrasts among the sisters. About a hundred yards from the main chapel was the room where Mass was held in the assisted-living wing. Some of the sisters who attended Mass there were residents of the separate St. Joseph's health-care wing and were severely disabled by strokes or Alzheimer's disease. Some of them could barely articulate a sentence, yet many managed to answer the priest with appropriate responses. Others silently fingered their rosaries. Well and able sat side by side with sick and disabled.

The door of each room in St. Joseph's had a picture of the sister with her name, so that new staff members could address each sister as an individual. Some doors had additional visual cues, such as a piece of colorful yarn tied to the handle, to help sisters find their way.

Most of the residents of this part of the convent weren't reading the Minneapolis *Star Tribune* or playing a mean game of Scrabble. Some slept sitting up in their wheelchairs or stared blankly into space. At times I would come upon a sister speaking a kind of unintelligible "word soup" and try to "talk" with her for a few minutes. Perhaps at least she would feel that I wished her well.

One day I came upon half a dozen of the less disabled sisters in a recreation room, where they were watching an old movie on television. "What are you watching?" I asked.

"Oh, just something," one of them answered in a pleasant voice.

I watched for a minute. "Looks like Lucille Ball is marrying Henry Fonda," I said. A few of the sisters murmured, "Oh, is that her?" or "That's Henry Fonda?" And then I added, "It's a Catholic wedding."

I was suddenly embarrassed by the absurdity of my comment. These women had spent the better part of a century as nuns. They would know a Catholic Mass when they saw one.

One of the sisters said, "Thanks for telling us," and we both laughed. But the expression on her face—one without irony, but with honest appreciation—caused me to ask, "Are you joking?"

She shook her head. "No," she said matter-of-factly. "I really didn't know."

⎯

As I drove back toward the Twin Cities, I would mull over my latest research ideas, only to toss them aside. The pressure from my department was growing less subtle. In a faculty meeting one of my colleagues archly referred to my work as "a study in search of a hypothesis," then laughed. Everyone knew you were supposed to start with a hypothesis and then look for answers.

Then I had a rendezvous with serendipity. Just as the three princes of Serendip of fairy-tale lore stumbled into discoveries as they traveled the world, my luck came to me as I strolled down a Mankato convent hallway and noticed a door ajar.

The door led to the Heritage Room, which had been closed on my previous visits, so I peered inside. Bookshelves lined the walls, as well as a glassed-in bookcase containing dolls of nuns dressed in different religious garb, chronicling the congregation's changing attire over the past two centuries. The size of a small den, the Heritage Room served as a sort of miniature museum about the history of the School Sisters of Notre Dame. What really interested me, however, was the office just beyond the Heritage Room.

The office belonged to the archivist of the Mankato convent, Sister Marjorie Myers. I introduced myself and then asked her about an adjacent room that, from the outside, resembled a bank vault. Sister Marjorie explained that the vault held the convent's historical records, and she offered to give me a tour.

The vault held several tall rows of old file cabinets. Neatly stuffed inside their drawers were lists of sisters who had taken vows, high school transcripts, photographs, autobiographies, death lists, and other detailed records describing the sisters' lives from childhood to late adulthood. For an epidemiologist, this sort of find is equivalent to an archaeologist's discovering an undisturbed tomb or a paleontologist's unearthing a perfectly preserved skeleton.

It was as though I had discovered a scientific study, started near the turn of the century, that closely followed a population over time, routinely collecting data and filing it away for later analysis. While most epidemiologists worry mightily about losing track of participants in a long-term study, these sisters belonged to their congregation for their entire lives. Better yet, many of the records in the file cabinets referred to women still living right down the hall. This meant that I could begin to design a study that supplemented this retrospective information with even more valuable prospective data, simultaneously looking backward and forward in time over their entire lives.

I had not found copper in Mankato. I had found gold.

2

The Last Nun Standing

My father had a store, and we, as girls, did the shopping for
the sisters. Their lives seemed so happy all the time, so I thought
I would like to live a sister's life.

—Sister Nicolette Welter

Many conditions that we now clearly recognize as diseases, such as cancer and osteoporosis, were once thought to be the result of old age. Fifty years ago, for example, most people believed that heart disease was simply part of nature's script for human beings. This was before Harvard epidemiologist Ralph Paffenbarger and British scientist Jeremy Morris noticed that occupation was strongly related to heart disease risk. Paffenbarger examined the lives of longshoremen in San Francisco and found that stevedores who loaded and unloaded cargo from ships had a lower risk of heart attack than their coworkers who sat at desks all day. Morris made a similar discovery: He found that London bus conductors who walked up and down the aisles collecting tickets in double-decker buses had a significantly lower risk of heart disease than the sedentary bus drivers.

Epidemiologists today continue in their efforts to untangle the skein of aging and disease. We still do not know exactly what drives the body's internal clock or how aging affects each organ in turn. My last study of the Seventh-day Adventists, which was ongoing during my early days at Mankato, addressed just such questions.

This analysis relied on a lifestyle and diet questionnaire completed by 19,586 Adventist women in 1976, together with the group's mortality records over the subsequent six years. We found that the later the age at natural (nonsurgical) menopause, the older the age at death. Every one-year increase in age at natural menopause was associated with a half-year increase in life expectancy.

More than any other organ, the function of the ovaries is driven by aging, with menarche starting a clock and menopause stopping it. The timing of the onset of menopause might indicate how fast the biological clock is ticking and provide a marker for the aging of other organs as well. Diseases, including some cancers, and other risk factors, such as smoking, also can bring on an early menopause. Thus an alternative explanation for our findings is that the ovaries are sentinel organs; reproductive fitness and health may simply be an indicator of overall health. Complicating the picture is the fact that it is hormonal secretions from the brain, the master organ, that start and stop the ovarian clock. Separating aging from disease is a difficult task, even when dealing with the ovaries, whose function is so controlled by age. It is exponentially harder to understand the effects of age on the brain.

Robert Butler, the founding director of the National Institute on Aging and author of a Pulitzer prize–winning book, *Why Survive? Being Old in America,* wrote the editorial that accompanied the publication of our findings in the *American Journal of Public Health.* "Alexander Pope, the English poet and student of man, said that the proper study of mankind is man, but the United States and other countries have devoted relatively few resources to studying the natural history of human phenomena, particularly aging phenomena," wrote Butler in his positive commentary about our work. Yet Butler ended with a cautionary note that I took to heart: "One is left wishing that the Snowdon, *et al.,* study were not just . . . a single photograph—but a longitudinal one—a cinematic record of changes throughout life."

Butler's comment was one reason I was so excited by my discovery of the Mankato convent archives. I realized that they might offer the kind of longitudinal view of aging that he had recommended. One of the first movies I ever saw was Walt Disney's *The Living Desert,* which used time-lapse photography to document changes that were imperceptible to ordinary observation. Perhaps I could splice together enough "snapshots" to watch a life unfold as vividly as one of Disney's desert flowers.

With the help of the Mankato archivist, Sister Marjorie Myers, I soon began poring over hundreds of historical documents. I also sought out Sister Nicolette Welter, the nun who had traveled a hundred miles to attend my first meeting with the sisters at Mankato. I was intrigued by her vitality, and I wanted to know more about her background. I hoped that by exploring the particulars of her life and comparing them with the lives of other nuns, I could elucidate some of the factors that increased the odds of growing old with an intact body and mind. Sister Nicolette proved to have marvelous recall for details of her life. She also taught me a great deal about what it meant to be a School Sister of Notre Dame.

Born in 1907, Sister Nicolette began life as Martha Welter, the fifth child of ten born to Peter Welter, a German immigrant, and Josephine Baltes, an American of German descent. The

Welters were leading citizens in the small community of New Market, Minnesota. Her father, Peter, owned the general store and a garage, and later served as the town's postmaster and undertaker. He was a devout Catholic, a generous man, and also the first in New Market to install indoor plumbing and electricity in his house. Sister Nicolette later told me that she would entertain the neighborhood children by switching the overhead light on and off. (Some of them were terrified by the flush toilet.)

The School Sisters of Notre Dame had a convent on the east side of town, and young Martha often delivered the mail there, usually with one of her little sisters in tow. During the mail drops, the nuns would give her a list of goods they needed from her father's store, but they also took the time to talk with her. Martha was enrolled at St. Nicholas parochial school in town, and she admired everything about the nuns, from their majestic black-and-white habits to the kindness they showed the townspeople.

By the time she was in the fourth grade, Martha knew that she wanted to join the School Sisters of Notre Dame. At age fourteen she could become an aspirant and enter the newly built high school for girls next to the provincial motherhouse in Mankato. But she hesitated to ask her parents. Mankato was far enough away that she would have to board at the school. As one of the older daughters, she was expected to help her mother with the housework and the younger children—not to mention that education beyond the eighth grade was often considered a needless luxury for a girl at that time. Most girls her age would work on a farm, or become a secretary or clerk, and then marry and raise a family.

Finally Martha asked one of the nuns to approach her parents on her behalf. The Welters gave their blessing proudly but sadly. They were a close-knit family, and in those days a girl who became a nun left the family circle forever. Home visits were usually allowed only when parents celebrated a golden or diamond wedding anniversary, when a brother performed his first Mass as a priest, or when her mother or father was dying. During Martha's last dinner at home, everyone at the table was in tears.

A young woman who feels called to become a School Sister of Notre Dame undergoes years of training to prepare her for the rigors of religious life. Beginning as an aspirant, she goes on to become a postulant (sometimes also called a candidate) and then a novice—all before professing first vows. These years are spent in taking high school and college courses, learning the traditions of the congregation, and devoting thousands of hours to service, reflection, and prayer. It is a long transformation, during which her commitment is tested and she grows into her new identity as a spouse of Christ.

Two years after arriving at the Academy of Our Lady of Good Counsel, Martha, then sixteen, joined the Mankato convent as a postulant. One week later she received an obedience from the mother superior: She was being sent to teach grade school in the state of Washington. (These obediences were called "bluebirds," because they were often delivered in a blue envelope and left at the sister's place in the convent dining hall.) Martha had no choice in the matter. Although the focus of the postulate was the candidate's own education, there was a desperate need for teachers in many of the Notre Dame schools. As an excellent student who had finished tenth grade, Martha was deemed ready for the job. A bright and energetic teenager, she saw her assignment to the Pacific Northwest as a "joy trip," an exciting and challenging adventure.

Martha left the next day for St. Paul, where she boarded a train heading west across the northern Plains. She arrived in Spokane after two full days of travel, and then took an eight-hour bus ride to the small post of Clarkston. The next morning, without even a day's rest, Martha began teaching the first, second, and third grades. She had no teaching experience and only a blessing from the mother superior to succeed. As she told me more than sixty years later, her strategy in the classroom was simple: "What I don't know, I will fake."

After teaching at Clarkston for a year, Martha returned to St. Paul to teach grade school. She continued her own education during the summers, although she did not receive her high school diploma until 1928. During this time, the mother superior granted her permission to attend her parents' twenty-fifth wedding anniversary. The momentous day was captured by a professional photographer, who clearly had a fine eye for composition. He placed Martha at the very center of the family group, where she stands serenely with her hands tucked into the sleeves of her long black dress, the graceful wings of her white bonnet streaming over the shoulders of her black postulant's cape.

August 13, 1925, was Martha's reception day, the day she became a novice and began—both symbolically and literally—to leave behind her old life. She would henceforth be called by her religious name, Mary Nicolette, in honor of her home parish, St. Nicholas. Her bonnet and cape would be exchanged for a white wimple that encased her face and fell almost to her waist; the novice's white veil would be pinned to the band that covered her forehead.

Near the end of the ceremony of investiture, the presiding bishop blessed these religious garments and sent the postulants into their new life: "Blessed be your departure from the world and more especially blessed your entrance into the City of God." At the chapel door, the postulants were met by their mother superior.

"My beloved daughters," she said, "the intention that you have in entering this convent should be no other than always to practice self-denial, to take up the Cross of Jesus Christ, and to follow Him."

"Reverend Mother, this is our intention, and we hope with God's grace to put it into practice."

She answered, "May our Lord bestow upon you the grace necessary to carry out this intention." She then presented each postulant with a crucifix. Each young woman also received her habit, her white veil, a breviary, a rosary, and a lighted candle. A wreath of roses and lilies, a symbol of purity and love, was placed upon her head.

And thus began a year of intense spiritual preparation. During that period, the novices had to maintain nearly complete silence, and their days were filled with prayer, contemplation, and instruction in the Holy Rule of the congregation. In Sister Nicolette's case, the novitiate actually lasted two years, since she spent another year in the field teaching before taking her first vows in 1927.

For many sisters, professing first vows was the single most powerful experience of their lives. On this day, they dedicated their lives to the mission of Jesus. Their white veil was exchanged for black, and they wore a crown of thorns, signifying their willingness to follow Christ's path.

The service came to its dramatic conclusion when the new sisters lay facedown in front of the altar in an act of submission and adoration. A large black shroud or pall was slowly drawn over the entire group, signifying the death of their old selves. When the pall was removed, they took their vows of poverty, chastity, and obedience and emerged from the chapel as brides of Christ.

Sister Nicolette took her first vows with fifteen other novices, and the day became an important anniversary that she and her classmates would commemorate for the remainder of their lives. Even as they took different paths away from the motherhouse to further their education and fulfill their work assignments, they would return periodically to renew their ties with one another. Finally retirement would reunite them, as it did for Sister Nicolette and her vows class of 1927, when she returned to Mankato from her parish post in Red Wing.

—

My growing knowledge about the sisters' lives, combined with the discovery of the archives, helped me at long last to find a focus for my work. During the next few years I would study the links between a sister's level of education and her mental and physical abilities late in life. According to the archival records, about 85 percent of the sisters had bachelor's degrees and about 45 percent had master's degrees—astounding statistics for any age group, let alone for women born in the early part of the century.

As early as the nineteenth century, British scientists had discovered a strong link between education and health—a correlation borne out by later statistics. Better-educated people lived longer, partly because they had a lower risk of a variety of diseases, from tuberculosis to heart failure. They even seemed to have a lower risk of Alzheimer's disease.

But how much of the difference was actually due to education and how much to the fact that until quite recently it was primarily upper-class people—with all their other advantages—who had access to advanced schooling? Maybe the real determining factors were related less to intellectual development than to socioeconomic status—differences in living conditions, diet, and access to health care.

Studying this link in the sisters would eliminate many of the confounding variables that plague epidemiologists. Income was not a factor, the sisters did not smoke, and they shared access to similar health care, housing, and diet.

Using funds from a small pilot study grant, I hired Sister Del Marie Rysavy, a young Mankato sister who was starting her doctoral work at the University of Minnesota. I also purchased three computers—IBM-XT clones, with what at the time were immense 60-megabyte hard drives. (Today we require well over a thousand times that capacity.) The science of epidemiology runs on data—mountains of it, combed and combined in every conceivable variation. My Ph.D. thesis had drawn on questionnaires filled out by nearly eighteen thousand Lutherans; my postdoc dietary studies on Adventists analyzed more than twenty-five thousand questionnaires. Now our team began entering the convent's educational records and death lists into our computers.

We also began developing the test protocols that would become one of the hallmarks of the Nun Study. Dr. Robert Kane, a highly respected gerontologist and the dean of the university's School of Public Health, had literally written the book (*Assessing the Elderly*) on performance-based testing. "Instead of asking a sister whether or not she can put on a sweater," he suggested, "ask her to put on one in front of you." He explained that it was natural for people to be too embarrassed or proud to admit to difficulties, and that they often exaggerated their abilities. Nurses' reports could be unreliable for the opposite reason: They tended to underestimate their older patients' competence.

With Sharon Ostwald, a geriatric nurse, we developed other methods of assessing both physical and mental function. We tested near and distant vision. We used a spring-loaded device to determine grip strength. We timed sisters as they opened and closed small wooden doors fitted with different latches. (It is difficult to take care of yourself if you can't button your clothes, open cupboard doors, or manipulate utensils.)

We also noted whether the sisters used mechanical aids such as canes and walkers, and determined whether they could rise from a chair. In one of the final physical tests, we timed how long it took each sister to walk six feet. Months later, when I tabulated the results, it astounded me that some of them had taken more than ninety seconds to complete this test. *Ninety seconds to walk six feet!* I realized how naive I had been about function in the elderly—and also how determined these sisters were.

Once when Sharon Ostwald and I were visiting the convent together, we walked into a room where a half dozen sisters were busily assembling stuffed animals. One elderly nun, who appeared to be in her late eighties, sat in a wheelchair stuffing cotton balls into a cloth giraffe. Osteoporosis had thinned her bones to the point that the vertebrae in her spine had collapsed, leaving her so bent over that her face was just above her knees. I froze; how could this woman function at all?

Sharon walked over to her, got down on both knees, and positioned her head within a few inches of the sister's face. "How're you doing, Sister?" she called out.

"Oh, just fine," the sister piped back in a surprisingly audible voice. "They've got me slaving away here for our holiday crafts sale. Forced labor, I call it." All the sisters in the room laughed—and a light went on for me. I should not be so concerned about disability. I should dive in and treat the sisters as the very individual human beings they were.

Our mental evaluation was rather crude compared to the battery of tests we developed later. We asked standard questions for determining orientation to time and place and basic memory (questions such as "Who is the president of the United States?" "What is the date today?" "What was your mother's maiden name?"). We also asked the sisters to solve some simple arithmetic problems.

My friend Sister Nicolette passed with perfect scores on all of our tests.

—

One morning twelve years later I had breakfast in the Mankato convent dining room with Sister Nicolette, then age ninety-one. We were joined by her biological sister Claverine, age eighty-four, one of the three younger Welter girls who had followed Sister Nicolette into the convent. Both Sisters Nicolette and Claverine had remained in fine health, and they strolled easily about the bright, pastel-painted room, serving themselves at the cafeteria-style counter. After we ate, I booted up my laptop to show the "sister sisters" a digitized version of the slide show that I had prepared about what had by then become known as the Nun Study.

A portion of my slide show, which I had presented at dozens of scientific meetings, included a description of Sister Nicolette and the fifteen other nuns who took their first vows with her. I began with the original photograph of the sixteen young women taken just before their reception day in 1925, when most of them were about eighteen years old. Just as she did in her parents' anniversary photo, Sister Nicolette stands tall in the center of the back row. Around her in perfect symmetry stand the other postulants, identically dressed, their white bonnets spilling down their shoulders and fastened by neat ties under their chins.

"Here is the fiftieth anniversary of first vows," I said as the screen filled with a black-and-white image of two rows of women, thirteen in all, who were now in their seventies. In 1977 only five of the sisters wore habits for their class picture; the others were neatly attired in modern clothes, a poignant reminder of how much the convent and the entire Catholic world had changed. Sister Nicolette's aquiline nose and jutting chin stand out more without her habit, although she still wears a black veil pinned to her hair. By this time she had earned bachelor's and master's degrees in education and had taught at nine elementary and junior high schools.

I then clicked my laptop's mouse and showed them the sixtieth-anniversary photo, taken when the sisters were in their eighties. This time the photo showed ten women, three of whom sat in the front row in their wheelchairs. Sister Nicolette again stood tall in the back at the center of the picture.

As we looked at the photo together, we talked about the fate of the six sisters who had died before it was taken, and about how the Nun Study already had begun to draw conclusions by comparing their histories with those of the women who had survived. Adding even more power to our analysis, ten more years had passed, and surely many more changes had occurred within this group of survivors, who would now be at least ninety.

"Go get Dr. Snowdon the seventieth-anniversary photo," Sister Claverine suggested. Sister Nicolette smiled knowingly and walked off to her room. She returned a few minutes later and put the eight-by-ten glossy on the table. "Here's the picture," she said.

The photo showed a solitary Sister Nicolette, standing and smiling at the camera, a corsage on her lapel and a pink glow to her face—the image of health and happiness. Although one other sister from her class was still alive for the anniversary, she suffered from Alzheimer's and had become too agitated to sit for the picture. That sister had died later in the year, leaving Sister Nicolette the sole survivor of her entering class of sixteen young women.

"Sister Nicolette is standing in every photo," said Sister Claverine. "She's the last nun standing."

—

Every stage of Sister Nicolette's long and healthy life adds to the "cinematic record of changes" that Robert Butler advocated. We can track her past through the data in the convent archives, and we can record her present and future through our ongoing mental and physical evaluations. We can analyze her genetic heritage, her childhood, her education, and her diet. We can, we believe, arrive at a clearer understanding of why she is the last nun standing.

Before we finished our coffee that morning, I put the

question to Sister Nicolette: Why did she think she had remained healthier than her classmates?

"I have an exercise program," she replied.

"What do you do?"

"I walk several miles a day."

"And when did you start this exercise program?"

"When I was seventy."

Sister Nicolette was right on target—as usual. Stroke and heart disease had been the two biggest killers in her class, and she had dodged those bullets. Exercise is one of the most reliable ways to preserve cardiovascular health, and its benefits apply at every age. All the walking she had done as a parish visitor in Red Wing had also helped to keep her mobile and to slow down the osteoporosis that might have thinned her bones.

In addition, Sister Nicolette's brain would have benefited. Exercise improves blood flow, bringing the brain the oxygen and nutrients it needs to function well. Exercise also reduces stress hormones and increases chemicals that nourish brain cells; these changes help to ward off depression and some kinds of damage to brain tissue.

Wherever my speaking schedule takes me, someone in the audience nearly always asks, "What is the first thing I should do to age successfully?" "Walk," I reply. "Walking is a great exercise for almost everyone." But I also say that the key point is to find some sport or activity that you truly enjoy, so that you will do it regularly—at least four days a week for the rest of your life. This not only protects your heart and bones; it also protects your brain.

And, as Sister Nicolette can attest, it is never too late to start.

3

Gray Matters

*Our congregation was founded to work with the poor and
powerless. Who's more powerless than someone with
Alzheimer's disease?*

—Sister Rita Schwalbe

On a winter's day in 1987 I sat in Emma Krumbee's
restaurant, halfway between Minneapolis and Mankato,
and spread out a series of scientific tables and charts to
review one last time. I finally had amassed enough data from my
studies of the School Sisters of Notre Dame to make a scientific
presentation that showcased our first findings and preliminary
conclusions. As I ate my pie made from apples grown in the now
snow-covered orchard behind the restaurant, I had one of those
fleeting moments where everything seems right: I had exciting
new data, a position at a top university, and an ongoing study
that seemed limitless. It also thrilled me that in a few hours I
would reveal my findings for the first time—and not to staid scientific colleagues, but to the School Sisters of Notre Dame
themselves.

Shortly after I arrived at Good Counsel Hill in the late

afternoon, some one hundred sisters who had agreed to participate in the pilot study filed into the meeting room to hear my talk. Although reporting new data to colleagues invariably gives my nerves a workout, today I was most concerned about the response of the sisters. Decades of teaching had honed their critical skills, and I worried that they would catch my every ungrammatical remark, inconsistency, and convoluted argument. Yet I did not worry enough about something more fundamental: the sisters' feelings.

The first investigation we did in Mankato examined the link between a sister's level of education and two aspects of aging: longevity and *active* life expectancy, or what might be called successful aging. (Most of us would say we want to live a long time—*if* we can also maintain independence in day-to-day activities.) I had seen dramatic differences among the sisters, some of whom were unable to feed themselves while others of the same age were still holding down full-time jobs, and I wanted to understand why these differences occurred.

Using the records in the Mankato archives that dated back to the early part of the century, we focused on a group of 306 sisters who would have been at least seventy-five years old in 1986 had they survived to that time. The longest-lived sister in this group had died at ninety-seven, before we began our study. The oldest living sister was ninety-four years old. In addition to compiling educational records, we assessed the mental status of the living sisters and whether they used daily nursing services or needed help with basic self-care tasks such as eating, dressing, and bathing.

Now I stood before the sisters and told them what we had found: that the sisters with a college degree had a much better chance of surviving to old age. They also had a better chance of maintaining their independence—without requiring nursing services or help with self-care tasks. Not only did the less-educated sisters have higher mortality rates, but their mental and physical abilities were much more limited if they did reach old age.

Of itself, this conclusion was not surprising, I said. I mentioned some of the earlier studies of education and longevity going back to the nineteenth century. I also pointed out that their own founder, Mother Teresa, had been way ahead of the scientists in recognizing the transformative power of education. The importance of our pilot study, I continued, was that it was so "clean"—without the variables that had confused earlier results.

As an example, I cited recently published research based on the celebrated Framingham data. Since 1948, the Framingham heart study had been following more than five thousand people in a small Massachusetts town. Much of what we now know about the relationship of coronary heart disease to hypertension and high cholesterol was first described in this landmark study. Earlier in 1987 the researchers had reported a strong connection between the level of a person's education and what they called "survival with good function." However, this data had many potentially confounding variables: A person who only finished grade school, for example, might be more likely to smoke cigarettes, earn less money, receive substandard health care, and live in shabby housing.

That is why it was so significant, I told the sisters, that the same results had emerged from our pilot study of the School Sisters of Notre Dame. They had similar lifestyles whether or not they graduated from college: Income was not a factor, they did not smoke, and they shared access to virtually the same health care, housing, and diet. Not only that, but the rich archives of the convent permitted another conclusion: The better-educated sisters had a lower risk of death at every age. In other words, the protective effects of education seemed to start early and last throughout life. This was further evidence that the connection to growing old gracefully could not simply be attributed to differences in health-related behaviors, income, or access to health care.

After my talk, I mingled with the sisters for a while. When the room had all but cleared, Sister Rita Schwalbe approached me. In the time since she had introduced me to the sisters during my first Mankato visit, she had become a good friend. "I know you meant well," she began, "but I thought I should tell you some of the sisters are upset about what you said."

"Upset?" I asked.

"It's the home service sisters," said Sister Rita, "the ones who didn't go to college." I knew that home service sisters did much of the domestic work at the convent. Now Sister Rita pointed out that many of the older home service sisters had had no opportunity for more than a grade-school education—usually at a rural one-room schoolhouse. A couple of them had told one of the elderly convent leaders that they felt terrible when they heard the statistics—they worried that they would not live as long and would need more help in their final years.

Months before, Sister Carmen had warned me about treating the sisters not as research subjects, but as people. I thought I had been conscientious about this. Sister Rita now had put me on notice that I had slipped. She was right, and the criticism stung. It was a mistake I vowed never to make again.

As I later discovered, the sisters were not alone in their consternation over these findings. Whenever I present them in public, I am challenged by my audience—especially because I have to admit that we still don't fully understand *why* education is so strongly linked to successful aging. I have heard many variations on "My mother never graduated from high school, but she is eighty-five, completely self-reliant, and active in her church" or, more sadly, "My father was a college professor, and he still got Alzheimer's."

In reply, I can only explain that epidemiology studies what is true of whole populations; it cannot predict the fate of individuals. And factors such as education—as opposed, say, to a vaccine—offer only a relative degree of protection. I sometimes point out that Volvos have a great reputation for safety—their structure reduces the chance of injury and death in an accident. Yet in spite of the good overall statistics, people do get injured and die in Volvos. I also emphasize the fact that most diseases develop as a consequence of a long chain of events. While we cannot change the past, we certainly can focus on lowering our risk now—by improving our diet or giving up smoking, for example.

In Alzheimer's disease, as in life, there are no guarantees.

—

At scientific conferences, researchers compete with each other for a chance to stand on a stage and present a short slide show that reveals their latest data. For a larger meeting, organizers may wade through a thousand or more submissions that briefly describe a project and its results. Half of these submissions typically do not make the first cut. Of the ones that do pass muster, maybe 20 percent of the researchers will receive ten or fifteen minutes to present their work. The other 80 percent receive a "poster" presentation slot, which consists of space on cloth-covered corkboards on which researchers pin up the pages of a paper that describes the details of their work. The researchers then stand in front of their posters and discuss their work with passersby.

When I submitted my Mankato data to a major scientific conference, the Gerontology Society of America's 1988 annual meeting, the organizers offered me a poster slot. Like most young researchers, I appreciated what amounted to an honorable mention, and I gladly made the trip to San Francisco to stand before my data and talk it up with some of the most respected gerontologists and researchers from around the world. But the turnout at my poster—and the poster session itself—fell far short of my expectations.

Except for researchers such as myself who were standing in front of their displays aching for attention, the conference seemed empty. It was like a poorly attended science fair for adults. Occasionally a handful of conferees would parade through the hotel ballroom, threading their way along the long rows of posters. Their modus operandi became predictable: walk slowly by each poster, give it a sideways glance, nod, and keep walking. It resembled the way a seasoned traveler determinedly navigates a gauntlet of peddlers in a tourist town, without stopping or talking to anyone. I couldn't help recalling that I'd had better audiences for my 4-H projects on chickens at the San Bernardino County Fair. The words of a colleague back in Minnesota echoed in my head. "Studying nuns?" he had said. "Whatever were you thinking?"

Finally around lunchtime a tall, authoritative-looking man in a well-pressed gray suit stopped in front of my poster and studied my data. "Jim Mortimer," he said in a deep, statesman-like voice, extending his hand.

Mortimer was director of geriatric research at the Minneapolis Veterans Administration Medical Center and worked only a few miles down the Mississippi River from me. It was a twist of fate that had brought us to San Francisco to meet. I knew that he had done highly respected research on both Parkinson's disease and Alzheimer's, and we spoke for a few minutes about the long-term studies that might be done with the sisters. He congratulated me on my poster, we shook hands again, and he walked away.

To my surprise, Mortimer returned an hour later to discuss more of my findings. I found myself talking animatedly, waving my hands as I described some of my ideas. Then an hour later he came back for the third time. "I think you've got some really good stuff," he said. "You're on to something." He nodded to himself while surveying my poster. "Ever considered studying Alzheimer's?" he asked.

When we returned to Minnesota, Mortimer and I kept our conversation alive, tossing around ideas about how the Nun Study could include the study of Alzheimer's disease. Mortimer had a particular interest in the hypothesis of "brain reserve," which directly tied in to my work with the sisters. The brain reserve idea suggests that the amount of disability seen in people with Alzheimer's does not simply reflect how much damage their brains have suffered from the disease. Rather, the way a brain develops in the womb and during adolescence may lead to a stronger or weaker structure. A stronger brain has more of a reserve, the theory holds, and symptoms may not appear even though Alzheimer's has done significant structural damage to the tissue. Mortimer described this stronger brain as one that was more efficient, with better processing capacity. This would enhance its flexibility or "plasticity," as the researchers put it. Thus it might be able to compensate by establishing new connections between nerve cells—in a sense, patching around the damage caused by Alzheimer's.

In his earlier work, Mortimer had been able to study the brains of a small number of his research subjects whose families had consented to an autopsy. If we could autopsy the brains of aging School Sisters of Notre Dame, he suggested, we would be able to address many mysteries of Alzheimer's. Maybe the association we'd found between education and mental function in elderly nuns indicated that the better-educated sisters had extra brain reserve and hence more resistance to the symptoms of Alzheimer's.

At first Mortimer's idea about brain autopsies struck me as

far-fetched, even repellent. Yet his musings intrigued me. If I wanted to reach deeper insights about the impact of education—or any other factor—on longevity, then I had to assess the threat that Alzheimer's presented. For all too many elderly people it was *the* major roadblock to aging successfully.

—

In 1901 the Hospital for the Mentally Ill and Epileptics in Frankfurt, Germany, admitted a fifty-one-year-old woman, Auguste D., who particularly caught the attention of a physican on staff, Alois Alzheimer. After developing an intense suspicion about her husband, the woman had begun behaving more and more bizarrely. She would hide objects. She would become lost in her own home. She sometimes would start screaming loudly, insisting that people were out to murder her.

When Dr. Alzheimer observed Auguste D. at the institution, he could not place her ailment into any known disease category. Her demeanor, he noted in a 1907 paper about the case, "bears the stamp of utter bewilderment." At times she would greet Dr. Alzheimer as though he were a visitor, and then she would excuse herself so that she could "finish her work." On other occasions she would scream madly, fearing that he wanted to cut her open. On still others she would send him away indignantly, implying he threatened her "honor as a woman." Dr. Alzheimer also noted that she frequently dragged her bedding around, calling for her husband or daughter. "Often she screams for hours in a horrible voice," he wrote.

By repeatedly approaching his patient, Dr. Alzheimer managed to complete a limited clinical evaluation. He found that Auguste D. confused lines when she read, repeated single syllables many times when she wrote, and often used odd phrases when she spoke (*milk pourer* for *cup*). "She clearly does not grasp some questions, and it seems that she no longer knows the use of certain objects," wrote Alzheimer. Auguste D.'s condition steadily worsened, and by 1906, the year she died in the institution, she "was totally dulled, lying in bed with legs drawn up, incontinent."

Perplexed by the case, Dr. Alzheimer autopsied Auguste D.'s brain. He focused on the outer layer, the location of the brain's gray matter—the part most associated with our human intelligence. In his landmark report, entitled "About a Peculiar Disease of the Cerebral Cortex," he noted that the autopsy revealed "a consistently atrophic brain"; damage and cell death had shrunk the tissue. He further noted that the nerve cells contained "a tangled bundle of fibrils." These, he observed, appeared "to go hand in hand with the storage of a pathologic metabolic product" around the nerve cells, which later researchers dubbed "plaques." Today, tangles and plaques are the two most important pathological features of what became known as Alzheimer's disease.

In addition to identifying tangles and plaques in Auguste D., Dr. Alzheimer further noticed atherosclerosis, or hardening of the arteries that fed her brain. This commonly causes strokes, which later would prove to play an important role in Alzheimer's disease.

Alois Alzheimer's groundbreaking work paved the way for future researchers. But in the late 1980s, when I first started discussing Alzheimer's disease in depth with Jim Mortimer, it surprised me that scientists still only had a flimsy handle on the degree to which plaques, tangles, and strokes contributed to Alzheimer's. Did everyone with plaques and tangles develop the symptoms of Alzheimer's? What caused these plaques and tangles to appear? Was it genes, or was it something in the person's upbringing or environment? Was aging the primary factor, or did many factors work together to bring on Alzheimer's?

When it came to Alzheimer's disease, there were more questions than answers.

———

Despite Jim Mortimer's enthusiasm, the future of the Nun Study looked dim as the 1980s drew to a close. My repeated attempts to win funding for the project had failed, and my department chair at the University of Minnesota had let me know as tactfully as possible that the faculty was unlikely to offer me tenure. Then in early 1990 I received a notice from the National Institute on Aging. My latest grant application, which proposed to study longevity and successful aging in nuns from all seven School Sisters of Notre Dame provinces in the United States, had been ranked in the ninety-sixth percentile—making it a sure winner.

Not only did the high score all but guarantee that I would receive funding, it also made me an attractive prospect to other universities. I soon had a job offer from, among others, the Sanders-Brown Center on Aging at the University of Kentucky Medical Center in Lexington. This was the second research institution established in the United States to study the process of aging, and it was already internationally known for its research on Alzheimer's disease. They offered great freedom to conduct my own research, and the atmosphere seemed blessedly cordial.

What clinched my decision to go to Kentucky was the reputation of the center's director, William Markesbery. As a neurologist, Markesbery had treated thousands of Alzheimer's patients, and he was known as the quintessential caring doctor. As a neuropathologist, he had also conducted autopsies on thousands of Alzheimer's brains. I explained to him my ongoing discussions with Jim Mortimer about expanding the Nun Study to include Alzheimer's disease and brain donation. Markesbery knew and respected Mortimer's work, and he backed our idea from the start.

The center's administrator, David Wekstein, was a physiologist who had launched the first medical study of centenarians in the United States. In his work with Markesbery he had also acquired vast experience with brain and body donation; he had recruited more than a thousand brain donors across the Bluegrass State. Until the Nun Study, however, the brain donations to the Center on Aging had come almost exclusively from people who had already been diagnosed with Alzheimer's. Markesbery and Wekstein recognized that this was akin to trying to determine the causes of automobile fatalities by studying only those who died in car accidents. If you really want to know how to prevent fatalities, you should also study those who walked away from the scene of the accident. The potential of the Nun Study was that we could examine many normal brains—and perhaps discover what had protected them from Alzheimer's.

Shortly after I arrived at the university in August 1990, serious discussions about branching into Alzheimer's began. At the time I did not know a plaque from a tangle, and Markesbery introduced me to his double-eyepiece microscope, which allowed us to examine the same slices of brain tissue simultaneously. Wekstein, meanwhile, schooled me in the particulars of how to ask for a person's brain, from the exact way to phrase my request to the whole gamut of concerns and fears the idea aroused in potential donors. From our first serious conversation on the topic, he made it clear that he saw me as an overly optimistic greenhorn.

One afternoon Wekstein and I met in his office, a charming mess that featured overstuffed bookshelves with slide trays stacked high atop them and a desk so cluttered with papers that it had no working space. The family photos that crowded the walls shared space with pictures of Wekstein standing next to the namesakes of the center—the father of former Kentucky governor John Y. Brown Jr. and Colonel Harland Sanders, the goateed and bow-tied dandy who started the fast-food chain originally called Kentucky Fried Chicken. Colonel Sanders had been sixty-five when he began his famous franchise business and seventy-four when he sold it—certainly a model of successful aging.

Wekstein raised his eyebrows high when I told him that I thought many of the elderly nuns at the seven main School Sisters of Notre Dame convents would agree to donate their brains. "They've devoted their lives to helping others," I said. "They have more altruism than the average person."

"Look, most of the sisters you're talking about haven't signed up for any study with you," said Wekstein, who rightly noted that I had yet to expand beyond the Mankato convent. "Even when we already have people in an Alzheimer's study, folks who clearly are motivated to help, 20 percent, at most, will agree to donate their brains. And that's with a lot of work. Lots of hand-holding and handshakes."

"Yeah, but the sisters are different," I protested.

"They probably are different," said Wekstein. "They probably are more altruistic than the average person. But they still may not want to donate their brains. The brain is not like other organs. People think of it as who they are—it contains their identity. It's loaded with meaning—personal, emotional, spiritual."

Jim Mortimer had become an integral part of this new study, and in one of our frequent phone conversations I relayed Wekstein's reservations. We arrived at a bold solution: Make brain donations mandatory for all participants in the Nun Study. The idea underwhelmed both Markesbery and Wekstein. "If this fails, you will have lost 80 percent or more of the sisters who otherwise might have joined," warned Wekstein. "That would also cripple the study on aging and disability that your new grant funds."

Then again, Wekstein and Markesbery recognized why Mortimer and I had floated this idea: If the majority of the sisters did agree to open their historical records to us, participate in regular mental and physical evaluations, and donate their brains for autopsies, we would have the makings of one of the most powerful Alzheimer's studies in the world.

4

---◆---

The Greatest Gift

As sisters, we made the hard choice not to have children.
Through brain donation, we can help unravel the mysteries of
Alzheimer's disease and give the gift of life in a new way to
future generations.

—Sister Rita Schwalbe

*T*he image of Michelangelo's *Last Judgment,* the master-
piece he painted on the rear wall of the Vatican's Sis-
tine Chapel, came into my mind one evening in
December 1990 as I paced the hallway outside the large meeting room at the Mankato convent. At the bottom left of the
painting, gray-fleshed corpses rise from their graves, called
from the dead to appear before Jesus Christ, who stands far
above at the center, his right arm raised in judgment. Then,
body and soul reunited, the resurrected are either carried joy-
ously by angels into heaven or dispatched, writhing and gri-
macing, to a fiery hell. This was the view of the afterlife that
had been seared into my consciousness at Sacred Heart grade
school, and I assumed as a child that on Judgment Day, you
would need all of your God-given body parts. Now, as I waited,
I replayed these images and wondered how the sisters would
respond to what I was about to propose.

I had made the trip to Mankato this snowy day with an entourage that included Jim Mortimer and Dave Wekstein. We ate dinner with the sisters, and afterward about 150 of the most elderly nuns at Good Counsel walked, wheeled, and shuffled into the meeting room. A large crucifix hung on one wall, and next to it stood a modestly decorated Christmas tree. Hissing radiators provided heat, and an uncovered fluorescent ceiling lamp in the front of the room brightly illuminated half of the women, most of whom wore a simple black veil, conservative modern clothes, and large eyeglasses. As the group settled themselves, I stood in front of them, nervously smiling and nodding to the many faces I had come to know well. Although I had talked with Sister Rita Schwalbe and the leaders of the Mankato convent about our plans, the potential participants in our study knew only that I was here to discuss a new research project. I worried mightily that I was about to jeopardize the many trusting relationships that I had worked so hard to build. I spotted Sister Nicolette sitting with her biological sisters. She nodded slightly and smiled to acknowledge my presence. Would she still be talking with me at the end of the day?

I began my presentation formally by thanking the sisters for meeting with me. "I am here to talk about Alzheimer's disease," I said. "It's one of the most dehumanizing diseases known to humanity—and one that has puzzled scientists for decades. Alzheimer's is a family disease, and by that I don't mean simply genetics. There are many victims besides the patient: Family members, friends, and caregivers are all deeply affected as they witness and attempt to cope with the relentless deterioration. You know this suffering in your own community," I pointed out, "but many families face it in painful isolation."

Many of the sisters nodded in agreement. This wasn't a theoretical issue to any of them.

"Even if Alzheimer's has never occurred in your family," I

went on, "it doesn't mean you won't get it. Old age is the most potent risk factor for Alzheimer's, and for those lucky enough to live into their nineties, about half will eventually develop the disease. And even if you escape, at some point you will likely help to care for a sister who has it."

Then I told them that they had the potential to alter the common view of aging, changing it from a time of despair to a time of hope. To do so, we needed more knowledge about the chain of events leading to Alzheimer's. By studying their lives, I said, we might be able to determine what causes Alzheimer's disease in some people and what could be done to prevent it in future generations. To move the study to the next level, I ventured, we also needed to study the brain.

I explained that plaques and tangles clearly played a role in Alzheimer's but that the fanciest devices scientists had built to peer inside a living human, including powerful CAT scan machines, could not see these microscopic entities. God encased the brain in an incredibly strong cranium, which protects it but also hides it from our view. So if we wanted to uncover the secrets of plaques and tangles, we had to examine the brain tissue itself, I said.

Then I took a deep breath and began to describe our new study. Sisters who joined would be asked to take a series of mental and physical evaluations each year. They would also be asked to donate their brain tissue after they died. (I stammered this out, hoping that gingerly asking for "tissue" rather than the brain itself would somehow seem less severe.) Finally I told them that they would still be able to have an open casket at their wake and that their friends and family would not be able to tell the tissue had been removed.

"Take as long as you like to think it over," I concluded.

Dead silence. And the silence, as silence does, grew louder with each passing second. Then I heard whispers in the back of the room. A few sisters over on one side began talking among themselves. The room slowly filled with a crescendo of voices, their volume and intensity replacing the shell shock that had occurred immediately after my request.

"Well, of course he can have my brain," I heard Sister Clarissa remark matter-of-factly. "What good is it going to do me when I'm six feet under?"

Sister Borgia Leuther, at age ninety-five one of the oldest convent residents, also spoke up. "He is asking for our help. How can we say no?"

As other heads nodded in agreement I glanced at Jim Mortimer, who was standing at the back of the room, smiling. I returned his smile and let out a sigh of relief. We had taken the first big step. And these women were on their way to making medical history.

—

In the weeks after the Mankato presentation we received a steady stream of consent forms from the sisters. Each form had to be cosigned by the convent's leader, who provided an important ethical safety check. The convent leadership also had power of attorney for the sisters.

I was aware of only some of the intense thought and prayer that guided many of the sisters in their decisions. I knew that official Church doctrine had approved of voluntary organ donation since the 1950s, but all Catholics were also taught in the catechism, as I had been, that the body was a temple of the Holy Spirit. Some sisters later spoke of how they resolved their feelings. "It is the spirit that is important after death, not the brain," said one. "At the resurrection, I believe our bodies will be glorified and perfect," said another. "We will have no illness and no physical defects. Resurrection does not depend on how our bodies are in the grave." Many sisters told me that their desire to help others had overcome their doubts. Another recalled that when her own sister had died in child-hood, her mother had allowed an autopsy because she thought it might help other families in the future.

In all, 90 percent of the 169 eligible Mankato sisters—we only recruited those who were at least seventy-five in 1991—initially consented to take part in the study. My coworkers and I now faced the task of determining how best to approach the other convents.

To make this decision, I turned not to scientists, but to sisters, recruiting Sister Rita and a handful of others to serve as collaborators. At Good Counsel we had already worked with the sisters for four years to build trust. Before we discussed our project with the School Sisters of Notre Dame at other convents, we similarly wanted to establish personal relationships. We knew that if we appeared to rush in, we might offend sisters who did not yet fully understand our aims or our practices. Sister Gabriel Mary Spaeth, a member of the provincial leadership team in Milwaukee, Wisconsin, quickly became an important member of our team. She had observed the Mankato meeting as her province's delegate, and now she agreed to help introduce us—and the importance of the study—to the sisters at Elm Grove, the large convent in a suburb of Milwaukee. Sister Marlene Manney from Mankato also volunteered to help us present the study at Elm Grove. Sisters Gabriel Mary, Marlene, and Rita would then travel with our team to the remaining five motherhouses on the same mission.

All three sisters stressed from the outset that the School Sisters of Notre Dame placed great importance on the spiritual concept of charism. They described this as "a gift of the Spirit given to an individual for the good of all." As Sister Gabriel Mary explained it, "Through baptism we share in the mission of Jesus. As School Sisters of Notre Dame, we live out that mission in the spirit of Mother Teresa of Jesus and Mother Caroline. Each sister carries the charism with her as she devotes her life to others. It's the spirit of our congregation." Sister Rita added that their charism included working with the poor and powerless. "Who's more powerless than someone with Alzheimer's disease?" she asked.

Elm Grove had a special significance for the congregation. In 1855 Mother Caroline Friess was traveling through the area to find a site for a convent when her horse stopped in the small village of Elm Grove and refused to move. She took this as a sign from God, bought forty acres from a local farmer, and began supervising the construction of the first building. Its castle-like design reflected the style of its benefactor, King Ludwig of Bavaria. Mother Caroline was buried at the convent after she died in 1892.

I was amazed when Sister Gabriel Mary led me through the halls at Elm Grove. Not only did she know the names of hundreds of nuns, but she had a personal query or comment for each of them. As one of the elected leaders of the province, she had spent the last four years working with the retired sisters, and from the way they greeted her, it was clear that they returned her love and respect. She flooded my mind with names and faces, and as I had at Mankato, I began spending day after day at the convent—often now joined by Dave Wekstein or one of our staff members.

I always attended Mass with the sisters before breakfast, and later in the day Wekstein and I would strike up conversations in the dining room or watch *Wheel of Fortune* or *Jeopardy* in one of the parlors, joining the sisters in their own game of trying to call out the answers before the contestants. I would walk with a sister around the convent's cemetery, listening to her stories about the past. I would chat with a sister while she sewed or made ceramics. Some, such as Sister Maria, immediately took a liking to me and invited me to their rooms to show me special mementos they had saved or crafts they had made.

Come Valentine's Day, I decided that we should hand-deliver a card to each sister. I came up with the idea after Dave Wekstein told me that he sent birthday cards each year to people who had enrolled in one of his Alzheimer's studies in Kentucky. On the flight from Lexington to Milwaukee, I handed Wekstein a stack of cards and asked him to sign them. I noticed that Wekstein, who has a serious wisecracking streak and usually has a comment about everything, was uncharacteristically quiet. At the end of the day he confessed to me that he'd thought the Valentine's cards were "one of the stupidest ideas I'd ever heard." But he flip-flopped when he saw how much the sisters—most of whom used to receive Valentine's cards from their students each year—loved our gesture.

The cards not only served as a terrific way to bond with the sisters, but also taught me an important lesson about Alzheimer's. In one of the convent's nursing wings, I handed a card to an eighty-five-year-old sister in full traditional black-and-white habit who was sitting slightly bent over in a wheelchair. She seemed quite disabled, and when she began to speak I could catch only a few disconnected words, and no meaning at all. After a few lame yesses and uh-huhs on my part, I pointed to the address on the back of the envelope. "That's where I am from, Sister," I said. "The Center on Aging."

The sister paused and looked up at me. "No," she said, her diction suddenly clear. "*This* is the center on aging." Then she laughed—and immediately went back to her private conversation.

This interaction—and others like it—convinced me that we have little idea of what a person with Alzheimer's disease can and cannot comprehend or of what is going on inside their heads. Just as surgeons have learned that patients under anesthesia can sometimes hear them, those of us who work with people suffering from Alzheimer's must at all times communicate with them as though they can understand.

At Elm Grove we changed our approach to the question of brain donation, bringing it up with small groups of sisters before we made our formal presentation. The presentation had evolved as well. It was now a team effort, with me leading off, followed by a staff member describing the mental and physical testing and Wekstein explaining why brain donation was so important to understanding Alzheimer's.

Sister Rita Schwalbe spoke last. She had recently returned to college and written a term paper on the ethics of doing research on the elderly. Now she told the sisters that she gave us high marks on that score, describing how much the Mankato sisters had enjoyed and taken pride in participating in the pilot study. She then spoke eloquently about how the study fit into the congregation's tradition of educating and helping others. But it was her final statement that I remember word for word: "As sisters, we made the hard choice not to have children. Through brain donation, we can help unravel the mysteries of Alzheimer's disease and give the gift of life in a new way to future generations."

During the next few years our team traveled the country to meet with the School Sisters of Notre Dame at convents in Baltimore, Maryland; St. Louis, Missouri; Chatawa, Mississippi; Wilton, Connecticut; Dallas, Texas; and Chicago, Illinois. Sisters Marlene Manney and Gabriel Mary Spaeth joined the Nun Study full time as field gerontologists, adding greatly to the sisters' trust in us. At each convent the reactions to our request mirrored the first meetings we had about brain donations in Mankato and Elm Grove: a long silence followed by resounding support for the project.

As the study grew, so did media interest. "Gift of Love" read the headline of a *Time* magazine article. *Life* magazine's cover story on neuroscience and the brain led with a description of the donation from the Mankato sisters. Frequently articles would quote sisters explaining that they had agreed to donate their brains because they wanted to help others after they died, and just as often they would make a joke about it, too. The St. Louis *Post-Dispatch* quoted Sister Loran Roche as saying, "We joke about all these Notre Dame nuns running around heaven without their brains." In the *Washington Post*, Sister Marie Xavier Looymans said, "I'll be up there, lookin' down while they're doing it. I won't feel it."

For those of us working with the sisters, these lighthearted quips were shadowed by more profound, and sometimes painful, reactions to our request—reactions that rarely made it into newspaper and magazine articles. It clearly caused turmoil for several sisters that they could not, in good conscience, join the study. A few sisters signed up and later withdrew, explaining that their families objected to the brain donation. "I want my last years of my life to be at peace with my family," a sister told Sister Gabriel Mary. "Every time we get together, they say, 'Are you still in that study?' " In Mankato in particular, the enthusiasm of the group's response led a number of sisters to sign up who later regretted the decision, dropping out by the first mental exam. Others told Sister Rita that they could not join because they believed, as one sister put it, that "I must return to God the way I came."

We explicitly did not pressure anyone to join—or to stay in—the study. I never wanted the sisters to feel as though they had to defend their decisions, nor did I want these women, who had devoted their lives to giving, to feel as though they were disappointing anyone by not giving in this instance. When a sister confided in me that she was sorry not to be participating, I would attempt to boost her spirits. "Sister," I would say, "keep us in your prayers. Then you will still be part of the study."

In all, 678 of the 1,027 eligible sisters enrolled in the brain donation program. That represented a phenomenal 66 percent rate of participation and held out the promise that the Nun Study would, as we had hoped, have the power to relocate the boundaries of knowledge about Alzheimer's disease and aging.

———

At 9:40 P.M. on June 26, 1991, Sister Angelus Schilling, a resident of Good Counsel Hill, died from a heart attack. Sister Angelus, eighty-nine years old and apparently in fine mental health, was the first of our brain donors to die.

I happened to be visiting the Mankato convent when Sister Angelus died, and I remember feeling both awe and fear when I heard the news. To my relief, we had established a process to retrieve her brain that did not involve me. Sister Rita contacted the night attendant at Landkamer's funeral home in Mankato, and within an hour after her death Sister Angelus' body was taken from the convent to Immanuel–St. Joseph's Hospital. At eight o'clock the next morning a pathologist made an elliptical incision around the top of Sister Angelus' skull, removed her brain, noted its weight in grams, and placed it in a one-gallon plastic container that held a solution of formalin. Over the next few weeks, the chemical would "fix" the tissue into a stable state. The pathologist stitched her scalp back together and returned Sister Angelus' body to the funeral home.

Sisters from Good Counsel then came to the mortuary to dress Sister Angelus in her habit and veil and prepare the coffin for viewing. During the wake, as Sister Rita told me later, many of the sisters observed the open casket with intense curiosity. They were clearly looking for scars or any other sign that her brain had been removed. There were none that they could see. "My, does she look nice," one sister discreetly commented to Sister Rita. "She looks so natural."

Two weeks later the hospital sent Sister Angelus' brain via UPS to the Center on Aging. I had never gotten to know Sister Angelus personally, and when the box arrived, I couldn't help being thrilled: It represented so many years of hard work—and so much potential for future research. Dave Wekstein, the veteran of hundreds of organ donations, watched my reaction intently. "Don't get so excited," he said. "Remember, somebody died."

5

A Tale of Two Sisters

*The prospect of having to start all over again in a new land
suddenly seemed frighteningly unrealistic. My fragile self cried
out in self-pity, "I am too old; it is too late!"*

—Sister Dolores Rauch

Town by town, the Nazi takeover of German society in
the 1930s was carried out through intimidation, ar-
rests, torture, and murder. One of the many targets of
their campaign was religious education. Many Catholic
schools were closed; religious curricula were prohibited;
would-be teachers were instructed to drop their religious affil-
iation and join the Nazi party; and Nazi-designed courses were
imposed to inculcate racism, nationalism, and militarism.

In the face of the Nazi threat, the American provinces of
the School Sisters of Notre Dame offered to take in any of
their German sisters who wanted to emigrate. When word
of this offer reached the Munich motherhouse, sixteen
prospective novices declared their intention to leave. And
then, one by one, their resolve weakened; many spoke no English, and they worried—with reason—that they might never

see their families again. So it was that on August 26, 1937, only two novices, accompanied by an older sister, boarded the steamship *Deutschland* in Hamburg, bound for New York.

The two young novices kept their own company during the eight-day journey. They felt awkward in their new habits and veils, which they had received only shortly before the trip, and hesitant in their new role as sisters. They also had strict orders not to discuss German politics with anyone, as rumor had it that some of the passengers were Nazi spies. In keeping with the customary restrictions of the time for novices, the young women maintained a discreet detachment from each other, too, never sharing private thoughts about this momentous leave-taking. To pass the time, they sang German songs—a favorite, one of them remembered later, was "Goodbye, Dear Homeland."

They disembarked at Ellis Island on a muggy September morning and then were driven from Battery Park through Manhattan to a convent on Ninety-fifth Street. More sisters had arrived on another ship, and before the end of the day the two novices were crowded into a station wagon with three other young women, plus a mother superior, for the twenty-six-hour trip—straight through—to Milwaukee, Wisconsin.

Nearly sixty years later, the wonder of that trip remained with them: the wide rivers with incomprehensible Indian names, the long ribbons of highway, the cities clogged with industry, the empty prairie that seemed to stretch on forever. Now and again, gently rolling hills and farmlands reminded them of home. The car had no radio, so again they sang their German songs. On September 5 they finally stopped moving.

Although the young sisters were used to sleeping on thick featherbeds, the sight of a convent room filled with thin cots delighted them. For the first time in ten nights, their beds would not be moving under them. Tired as they were, however, they lay awake, their minds racing, long after the other sisters in the room had fallen asleep. As the convent filled with the Great Silence of the evening hours, they listened to the strange new American sounds outside the window until their excitement finally gave way to exhaustion.

———

One of the two "German novices," as their American sisters called them, was Sister Maria, who had befriended me on my first visits to Elm Grove. Intrigued with the bits of her story that she told me, I began to reconstruct her history from the records carefully stored in the convent's archive. At Mankato I had made a discovery that was to have enormous consequences for the Nun Study: Nearly every sister's file included one or more autobiographies that she had written after joining the congregation.

The School Sisters of Notre Dame tradition of autobiography might be said to have begun with Mother Caroline Friess, the first leader of the American sisters. During the five decades she spent traveling through the young nation, she recorded her journeys in extensive journals and hundreds of letters. Her writing is vivid with feeling and telling detail; whether she was documenting the evils of slavery or recounting her narrow escape from a Mississippi steamer that exploded in midriver, she displayed a true gift for storytelling.

This said, the congregation's records do not explain why, on September 22, 1930, Mother Mary Stanislaus Kostka, the Superior for North America, sent a letter to all the convents requesting that each novice write an autobiography before she took her vows. The letter called for a short sketch of their life:

This account should not contain more than two to three hundred words and should be written on a single sheet of

*paper. . . . Include place of birth, parentage, interesting
and edifying events of childhood, schools attended, influences that led to the convent, religious life, and outstand-
ing events.*

Since there are earlier autobiographies on file, Mother
Mary Stanislaus may have recognized a legacy in the making.
She may also have reasoned that the novices' autobiographies
would give her insight into the background the young sisters
brought to the work ahead of them. Once after I described
these autobiographies at a seminar, a psychiatrist approached
me and said, "I'll bet the autobiographies were an attempt to
assess the younger sisters' mental abilities and aptitudes. I
think the mother superior was really acting like a neuropsychologist." In 1930, standardized intelligence and personality
testing was still in the future, and, of course, even today many
high school seniors agonize over personal essays on their college entrance applications.

There were hundreds of autobiographies in Milwaukee
alone, most handwritten in the graceful script inculcated by
generations of teaching nuns. Not only could I reconstruct a
sister's educational and medical history from the records kept
by the congregation, but I could glimpse her childhood and
the early influences that had shaped her mind and personality. As I read Maria's autobiography, written in 1938, her early
life came into focus in a series of vivid snapshots.

On January 30, 1913, a tailor's wife in an ancient Bavarian
town gave birth to twin girls. The babies were so fragile that
they were baptized that same night in a private ceremony at
the parish church. Baby Johanna would grow up to become
Sister Maria. Her sister Magdalen died before the next day

dawned. Johanna's parents later would say that her lively disposition had taken too much life from her twin.

Young Johanna's rambunctious nature earned her the nickname Rumpela—which means something like "whirlwind." In one of her escapades she was returning from an errand for her father with her cousin Heinz riding in the delivery cart. She pushed the cart so hard that he lost his grip, sailed into the bushes, and broke his leg. At six she entered a grade school conducted by the School Sisters of Notre Dame and promptly announced that she, too, would become a nun. In her autobiography Sister Maria recalled, "Nobody would believe me." "You have enough life for two boys!" her teacher said to her one day.

Sister Maria described the years growing up with her three sisters and two brothers as "very happy," and the presence of the Church in her life became "more firm" after she took her first communion at the age of ten. When she turned thirteen, she read the autobiography of St. Thérèse of Lisieux, a French Carmelite nun who was called "the Little Flower" and the patroness of the missions. "Like many others I dreamt very often that, when I was grown-up, I would go to Africa to teach the children there," Sister Maria's own autobiography explained.

Later that year Johanna moved to Weichs, a city near Munich, to attend the teacher training school conducted by the School Sisters of Notre Dame. But her life soon took a dramatic turn for the worse. Her father, a veteran of the Great War, became gravely ill. His illness forced Johanna's mother to take complete responsibility both for the family business and for the children still at home. Her father suffered for the next four years, which "broke the strong constitution of my mother." By the time he died, in 1930, Johanna's mother had herself become ill and would become more and more incapacitated until her death four years later.

Johanna continued with her training as a teacher and a

nun, and for more than two years she taught her own second- and third-grade classes. Nevertheless, these hard times took their toll. "These sad events in our family . . . served to change my former liveliness into greater seriousness," her 1938 auto- biography notes. Maria was an orphan when she boarded the *Deutschland* and stepped into the unknown.

"What gave you the courage to leave?" I once asked her. She replied, "I knew God would provide all that I needed in Amer- ica."

—

After Sister Maria's death I began using video clips of her mental examinations as part of the presentation I gave about the Nun Study at scientific conferences, colleges around the country, and community centers, where I could meet with people who cared for loved ones with Alzheimer's. For every audience, Sister Maria's image puts a real human face on Alzheimer's: While the videotapes show the progressive loss of her short-term memory and orientation in time and place, they also demonstrate that some of the most beautiful parts of her brain and mind were still intact. Regardless of her mental and physical difficulties, she remained very much human.

In the fall of 1997, I was giving such a lecture at Mount Mary, the Milwaukee college owned by the School Sisters of Notre Dame. Because Sister Dolores Rauch was both a partici- pant in the Nun Study and a professor at the college, she was asked to greet me before my presentation. As was usual with the sisters, she was extremely polite and affable, but it was the energy of her intelligence that impressed me the most. She looked directly in my eyes as we spoke, and the wheels in her head seemed to turn with deliberate precision with every ques- tion I posed to her.

After I finished my talk, Sister Dolores approached the lectern with an excited look on her face.

"Dr. Snowdon, I was the other nun!" she said.

"Excuse me?" I said.

"You see, when I heard you talk about Sister Maria, I thought to myself, 'Oh, my goodness! I was the other sister who came with Maria from Germany!' "

Her words took a second to register. During all of our conversations, Sister Maria had never told me the name of her traveling companion. Now here she was before me, a participant in the Nun Study. I was stunned at the good fortune of this discovery. Even though, as an epidemiologist, my focus is on comparing large groups, I found it irresistible to trace the parallel lives of Sisters Maria and Dolores. It was like finding the long-lost survivor of a car crash who could tell me the reasons she survived and her fellow passenger did not.

—

Like Sister Maria, Sister Dolores was born in Bavaria, and her childhood was shaped by the Great War. Her father, too, was a veteran, and since Dolores (or Barbara, as she was christened) was born in 1916, while he was still in military service, her mother teased her by telling her she had inherited his warlike qualities.

Despite the hardships of war and its aftermath, Barbara's recollections of her life growing up had an almost romantic quality. While her father was fighting in Bulgaria, her mother had kept the family farm running with the help of a few maids and a prisoner of war. The Rauch family lived in an ancient stone farmhouse, and sometimes hungry strangers would come to the door begging. Her mother always found food to share. Barbara still remembered the price of admission at the first puppet show she attended: one egg.

As the sixth of eight children, Barbara held her own among her siblings and nearby cousins. She was proud of her status as a tomboy. "I was the only girl the schoolboys invited to go sledding," she once told me with obvious pleasure. Her mother referred to Barbara as her "second son."

Again like Maria, Barbara decided on her profession on the first day she attended school. "I am going to be a teacher," she declared. Later that year Barbara would become captivated by a missionary priest who visited her class. The priest enthralled seven-year-old Barbara with his tales of the far-off continent of Africa, where children had no schools or clothes and often went hungry. After he finished his talk, he fished through his bag and removed a figurine of a boy, his hands clasped in prayer, kneeling on a green painted box. "This African child is praying for help," the missionary explained. "Would you like to assist God to answer his prayer?"

Barbara nodded, along with her thirty other classmates. The children lined up, each holding the coin their teacher had told them to bring for missions day, and made a procession to the collection box. Barbara watched, fascinated, as the boy's head bobbed a thank-you for every coin dropped through the slot at his knees. From that moment she began to dream of going to Africa one day as a missionary teacher.

Barbara excelled in school, and her third-grade teacher often asked for her help with the younger children, calling her *Vizelehrerin*, or assistant teacher. One winter evening the assistant pastor of their parish stopped by the farmhouse. Barbara and her siblings had taken over the large kitchen table to do their homework. Her mother sat in a rocker, a new baby in her arms.

"Mrs. Rauch, you have seven daughters," the young pastor said. "Have you thought about letting one of them enter the convent?"

"This is not for me to decide," Mrs. Rauch said. "The decision is their own."

"I am not going to the convent!" declared the eldest daughter, marching out of the room.

"I'm not, either," insisted the next in line, who also left the room, followed by the third.

Barbara, barely nine, watched in wonder. The pastor turned to her. "What about you?" he asked.

"I'm going to be a teacher," Barbara said resolutely.

"But you could become a sister teacher," the pastor suggested.

"How can I become a sister teacher?" she replied. "I've never even seen a sister."

Barbara forgot about the conversation until shortly before the beginning of the next school year, when her mother received a letter from the government approving Barbara's transfer to a school taught by the School Sisters of Notre Dame. Her mother seems to have had a remarkable respect for her daughters' independence, and she stressed that Barbara did not have to make the change. "But it is a better school, and you will learn more."

"Then I'll go," Barbara immediately replied.

Although Barbara had to rise at five-thirty each morning and walk nearly an hour through the forest to reach her new school and attend High Mass, she loved the beauty and peace of the woods, and her religious conviction grew. The next year she came home from school one day and announced to her parents: "I love school, I love learning, and I love Jesus. I want to be a priest." But not just any type of priest. She wanted to be a Jesuit, free to spend the rest of her life immersed in both intellectual and spiritual pursuits.

At the end of seventh grade, with the help of her pastor, she filled out an application to study at an institute run by the Holy Ghost Sisters, a congregation with missions in Africa. To

Barbara's dismay, her father put his foot down. "Child," he said, "you are too young to make such a decision. We love you too much to let you go so far away. Besides, there is enough work to do right here in Germany—if you *must* become a sister."

Again at her pastor's suggestion, Barbara enrolled in a six-year combined high school and college program at a boarding school conducted by the School Sisters of Notre Dame. Barbara still did not intend to join the congregation; she was after a teaching credential. Yet she developed a profound respect for the spirit of the sisters and their devotion to education. Now she faced a painful dilemma: If she joined the congregation, she would have to abandon her dream of Africa, since the sisters did not work on that continent.

Barbara sought the advice of her confessor. "It seems to me that God is calling you to the School Sisters of Notre Dame," he said. "If and when God wants you to serve in Africa, you will receive an unmistakable sign." So in 1936 Barbara Rauch became a postulant with the School Sisters of Notre Dame.

Her first assignment was as assistant to the principal at a public elementary school run by the congregation. As part of her continuing training, she had to attend government-run workshops once a month. At one of these meetings near the end of the 1937 school year, the supervisor read an official letter that advised all would-be teachers to drop their affiliations with religious communities and join the Nazi party.

"The letter was pure Nazi propaganda, dripping with venom and directed toward religion in general and sisters in particular," Sister Dolores wrote in her lengthy and richly detailed memoirs, which she shared with me. "Anger, frustration, and fear shook my very being. I took the long way back to the convent. Walking through the quiet park area, my mind cleared and my heart vowed, 'You will never get me into your ranks, no matter what the consequences might be.' "

Barbara went to her father and asked whether she could accept the offer made by the American provinces to take in German members of the congregation who wanted to emigrate. Absolutely not, he said. Although he despised the Nazi regime, Barbara's father, like many Germans, believed that Hitler would never last. A few weeks later a pastor in a neighboring town who had spoken out against the Nazis disappeared. "I really should have let her go," Barbara's father confided to her mother, who promptly passed on the news of his change of heart.

On August 9, two weeks before she boarded the *Deutschland* for the United States, Barbara was received as a novice and took the religious name of Dolores, with all its overtones of suffering. Her parents came to the ceremony. She would never see them again.

After they arrived in America, Sisters Maria and Dolores spent their novitiate year at the Milwaukee motherhouse. Located in the center of the city, it occupied an entire square city block and was designed much like the Munich motherhouse, with offices, living quarters, and a chapel surrounding an immaculate inner courtyard, which offered a cloisterlike seclusion. But the motherhouse could not shield the sisters entirely from the social upheaval of the city. Anti-German sentiment permeated the United States, as Hitler had just taken the Sudetenland and would soon be invading Poland. Many Milwaukeeans of German descent stopped conversing in their native tongue; although many of the sisters at the motherhouse spoke German, they also made an effort to use English at all times.

This situation particularly affected Sister Maria, because she knew very little English and spoke with a heavy accent. Sister

Dolores, on the other hand, had studied English for five years in Germany. Her biggest problem was her British accent and vocabulary. "It took months before I could comprehend jokes," she told me.

The German sisters took classes together, including one with a speech therapist to help them master the subtleties of American English. Their report cards reveal that both women had sharp intellects, with their near-identical grades ranging from the high 80s to the high 90s. Yet their personalities differed dramatically, and they began to drift apart. A walk they took together stood out in Sister Dolores' mind decades later. "Dolores, you're always hopping all over the place," Sister Maria reprimanded. "Maria was very, very sedate," Sister Dolores recalled. "She was controlled and private." The girl nicknamed Rumpela seemed to have vanished.

Their autobiographies also strike a different note. Sister Maria's concludes with a dutiful account of her new life in America: "There amid dear companions and under the direction of kind Superiors we are preparing for our future occupation—to be teachers of Catholic Youth for the salvation of their immortal souls." Sister Dolores' essay ends in something close to poetry: "Dependence upon grace, I might call my former life; thanksgiving for this grace, I will choose as a motto for my future."

In August 1938 both sisters professed their first vows. The following month they received their "bluebirds," or teaching assignments. Then their lives split apart, and they would follow very different paths for the next half century.

—

Ill health dogged Sister Maria from the start.

Her first assignment was to teach a second-grade class at St. Joseph's School in Appleton, Wisconsin. Her vow of obedience meant that she accepted it without question, but the isolation and stress of her first year in America had taken its toll. On her first day of school Sister Maria suffered a nervous breakdown, and by all accounts it appeared to be an episode of severe depression.

At that time, a separate building in a wooded area of the Elm Grove property was set aside to care for sisters suffering with any kind of mental illness. Sister Maria stayed here for the next two months, during which time another German sister helped to bring her out of her shell.

She was able to remain at her next assignment—again a second-grade class—for four years, until a serious tooth infection in 1943 kept her from work for six months. Five years later she contracted tuberculosis and was treated at the TB sanatorium at Elm Grove, staying this time for four years. Upon her recovery Sister Maria returned to teaching, but she quickly had another nervous breakdown. After a psychiatrist advised her not to teach, she took a job in the tapestry room at the Milwaukee motherhouse, where she made and mended the priests' liturgical garments or vestments.

This was her assignment for the remainder of her working life, whether at the original motherhouse in Milwaukee or, after 1954, at its new location in Mequon. Her tuberculosis recurred, and she had two lung operations with long convalescences. She considered 1963 a red-letter year, as the province sent her to Rome and then to Germany, where she visited relatives for the first time since 1937. She retired from her seamstress job at Mequon in 1982.

When I met Sister Maria in 1991, she lived at the Elm Grove retirement facility. I knew from her first mental exam, in which she could only recall four of ten words, that she had problems. But Rumpela seems to have returned a bit to lighten her old age, and Maria was so witty and charming that her rapid decline during the next few years surprised and saddened me. In the last test we gave her, nine months before her death on January 26, 1996, she could not even repeat the phrase "no ifs, ands, or buts." I hardly recognized this woman whose company I had grown to cherish. And she showed no signs of remembering me.

—

As I traced Sister Dolores' history, I was struck by how much her life had diverged from Sister Maria's.

Determined to prove herself in her new homeland, she had thrown herself into her studies and into her job as a teacher. But she too struggled with loneliness. Throughout the war, her only contact with her family was through the Red Cross, which twice a year would forward a letter containing no more than twenty-five words. One letter contained the news that her beloved only brother had died in combat at the Russian front. Then in 1944 the Red Cross notified her of her mother's death—which had taken place a year earlier. These losses devastated Dolores, but she viewed them as God's will. Her ability to go on strengthened her belief that with God's help she could survive anything.

During the next two decades Sister Dolores was assigned as a teacher and then a principal to the congregation's schools scattered throughout Wisconsin. Like most sisters, she taught nine months a year and attended college during the summers. She earned her bachelor's degree in 1945, when she was twenty-nine years old, and her master's degree in 1960, at age forty-four.

When she was forty-seven years old, Sister Dolores became a professor of elementary education at Mount Mary College in Milwaukee. Her friends predicted that she was "stuck for life." But then the college lost its geography instructor, and the president asked Sister Dolores whether she wanted to train to teach the subject. Excited by the idea of exploring a new field, she went back to school again, earning an M.A. in geography at age fifty-one and a Ph.D. at fifty-five.

By the early 1970s the School Sisters of Notre Dame had extended their work to Africa. *That's where I should be*, Sister Dolores told herself. She began speaking about her dream with her friends. "That's my continent," she would tell them. "I have been waiting to go there since I was knee-high." But Sister Dolores reluctantly agreed with the reaction that typically greeted her: She was too old.

Then in June 1983, at age sixty-six, Sister Dolores took part in a religious renewal program at the congregation's world headquarters in Rome, where she attended a presentation by a sister who had been working in Africa. As she was leaving, Sister Dolores happened to pass Sister Mary Margaret Johanning, the congregation's general superior. "That's my continent!" Sister Dolores blurted out as she walked by.

"You want to go to Africa?" Sister Mary Margaret called after her. "Are you serious?"

Sister Dolores turned back. "I have always wanted to serve in Africa, but it is too late now," she said. "I am too old."

"That is not necessarily so," Sister Mary Margaret replied. "Think and pray about what you would do if you were given a chance to work in Africa. I will see you tomorrow about your answer."

In Sister Dolores' memoir, she described how the possibility of working in Africa suddenly overwhelmed her. "I thought of my work at the college, which I loved, my friends, my family, my health situation—of letting go of all I had built up during a lifetime," she wrote. "The prospect of having to start all over again in a new land suddenly seemed frighteningly unrealistic. My fragile self cried out in self-pity, 'I am too old; it is too late!' " But then she saw a glimmer of light in her imagination that grew brighter and brighter. God, she concluded, was sending her the sign that her confessor had spoken of forty-eight years earlier.

Sister Dolores soon received word from Rome that she was being assigned to a post in Kenya. "It was like winning the lottery," she said.

—

Sister Dolores arrived in Kenya in 1984—two years after Sister Maria had retired from her job in the tapestry room. The local bishop dispatched her to South Nyanza, near the northeastern edge of Lake Victoria. He asked her to study the starvation that was occurring in the region and to devise a remedial program that the local residents could maintain on their own. After assessing the situation, Sister Dolores realized that the villagers had overharvested the trees without planting new ones and that this, combined with recent climate changes, had caused desertification and crop failures.

To combat this problem, Sister Dolores started a reforestation project called Community Mobilization Against Desertification. She kicked off her fund-raising drive at the Ford Foundation office in Nairobi, refusing to leave until she saw a project officer. The Ford Foundation had never funded a project in Kenya run by a religious group, but after Sister Dolores doggedly pursued them for two years, the philanthropy came through with money for her endeavor.

In 1992 Sister Dolores, now age seventy-six, returned to Mount Mary College for a sabbatical year, which she spent teaching herself about computers. That year she joined the Nun Study and scored high marks on her first mental examination.

Sister Dolores was not available for her second examination in 1994, as she had returned to Kenya to steward the reforestation program. My colleagues and I debated whether to drop her from the study, because our protocol required complete records. However, we realized that it would have been ridiculous to eliminate someone from the study for being too able-bodied and busy. Sister Dolores became the first nun that we allowed to skip an exam.

In 1996, Sister Dolores, then eighty years old, said goodbye to Kenya. South Nyanza had become greener, and the farmers had developed their own programs to solve their common problems. Despite all that remained to be done, Sister Dolores had lived out her childhood dream of helping Africa—one that she had all but conceded would never be fulfilled.

After she returned, she took her second Nun Study examination and had a near-perfect score. In stark contrast, 1996 was the year that Sister Maria, weakened by Alzheimer's, contracted pneumonia and died within a few days.

——

Many people still believe that, as we age, our minds wear out, and that if we live long enough, we will inevitably become demented. This is a myth. Aging does increase the risk of developing Alzheimer's, which helps explain why Sister Maria did not suffer from the disease until her eighth decade. But clearly Sister Dolores' mind did not deteriorate after eighty years of use. What, then, explains their different fates?

In the world of epidemiologists, anecdotal evidence—like the parallel lives of Sisters Maria and Dolores—is deeply suspect. Stories about individuals can make for persuasive tales, yet not reflect reality. The more we know about Alzheimer's, the more complex and multidimensional it seems, with roots that go back to childhood. Only studying large groups can help untangle all these influences.

Such studies suggest a long list of factors on which we might compare Sisters Maria and Dolores. For example, Jim

Mortimer and other researchers have shown that head trauma is a risk factor for Alzheimer's—but this factor is missing from both sisters' histories, as far as we know. We are also limited in our ability to trace genetic influences. Neither Sister Maria's nor Sister Dolores' parents developed Alzheimer's disease, but this may simply reflect the fact that they died relatively young. And while a few Alzheimer's-related genes have been identified, current thinking is that a dozen or more—perhaps many more—may work in tandem to increase either susceptibility or resistance to Alzheimer's.

Certainly being female increased the risk for both women. Women as a group live longer than men, but this does not explain the entire difference in risk. It appears that many men who live longer than average for their gender are "hardy" in some way—they are unusually resistant to many diseases, including Alzheimer's. In the general population of women, differences in reproductive history and in the use of estrogen after menopause are thought to affect the risk of Alzheimer's, but, again, these factors do not apply to Sisters Maria and Dolores. The Nun Study has not addressed the question of whether estrogen replacement reduces the risk of Alzheimer's, because almost none of the participants used it. We, like most clinicians, await the results of ongoing studies now being conducted by the National Institutes of Health, particularly the Women's Health Initiative, a large-scale clinical trial. Within the next few years, this study should provide the best available data on whether estrogen replacement can reduce the development of memory impairments and dementia in women sixty-five and older.

One clear difference between Sisters Maria and Dolores is in education. Our own pilot study found a clear link between higher education and healthy function in later life. And most of the large studies throughout the world have found links between lower levels of education and Alzheimer's. Although the two nuns received nearly identical education through their early twenties, their experiences diverged sharply after their first year in the United States. Sister Maria worked in elementary schools off and on, but spent most of her career as a seamstress. Her hopes of completing a master's degree were derailed by her many bouts of illness. Sister Dolores moved up the academic ladder throughout her career, from elementary school teacher to principal to college professor. Along the way she earned a bachelor's degree, two master's degrees, and a Ph.D. These differences in education dramatically influenced how they lived their lives, but they may have had little, if any, effect on their Alzheimer's risk. Most studies show increased risk only for those without any college education. (Nun Study conclusions are actually limited in this regard because we have so few participants at lower educational levels.)

Another pronounced difference between the two sisters was in their family upbringing and environment. I was curious to know more about Sister Maria's family, and in 1999, at my request, Sister Dolores contacted a nephew of Sister Maria's who lived in Germany. He had gotten to know his aunt when she visited in 1963, and he turned out to be a wonderful source of family lore.

The account he later sent me, via Sister Dolores, was much darker than Sister Maria's youthful autobiography. "Maria herself," he wrote, "has always emphasized that they had a hard childhood and that her father was very strict, especially after his return from World War I with shattered nerves." His uncle Heinz (the cousin whose leg Sister Maria accidentally broke) had told him stories. While Heinz was recovering from his broken leg, a neighbor brought him a cake. This enraged Sister Maria's father for some reason, and he threw the cake down the stairs. Uncle Heinz also had a story about Sister Maria's birth. According to him, her mother actually *prayed* that God would take one of her twin daughters, so overwhelmed was she by having two newborns to care for simultaneously. (I recalled with shock that her parents had told young Johanna that her own liveliness had taken "too much life" from her sister.)

These are only snapshots, of course, but they form a sharp contrast to Sister Dolores' family, where her mother seemed to enjoy her large brood, and her father tried to keep his daughter close—until her safety was threatened.

Such family circumstances may have played a role in Sister Maria's depression, which was evident soon after she arrived in America as a young novice, as well as later in her life. Among older adults, depression occurs more often in Alzheimer's patients than in healthy controls. (Depending on which study you believe, between 15 and 40 percent of Alzheimer's patients are depressed.) However, the nature of the link between depression and Alzheimer's is unclear. Is depression a risk factor for Alzheimer's? Or is depression an emotional response to the losses caused by Alzheimer's?

Several major studies suggest that depression predates the onset of Alzheimer's and constitutes a distinct risk factor. One analysis compared people with Alzheimer's with a control group of people who did not develop the disease. After combining data from four studies, they concluded that people who had been depressed *before* being diagnosed with Alzheimer's had a 1.8 times higher risk of developing the disease. This near doubling of risk held up even when the researchers evaluated people whose history of depression began ten years or more before their Alzheimer's was diagnosed.

There is no doubt that treating depression in Alzheimer's patients can result in improvements in their mental, social, and physical functioning. And since depression is also an important risk factor for coronary heart disease and other chronic diseases, it may have played an additional role in Sister Maria's premature death—premature at least by the standards of our long-lived nuns.

We may never know the precise reasons why Sister Maria developed Alzheimer's disease and Sister Dolores was spared. But since both sisters joined the Nun Study, their histories are now part of a powerful database created to address these perplexing questions in detail. As the Nun Study began to peer into the brain itself, entirely new landscapes came into focus—and we discovered that we still had surprising things to learn from Sister Maria.

6

Amazing Brains

This will be great. I was born in Kentucky, and now my brain
will be going back there.

—Sister Carlene Roberts, Chicago province

*I*t's been a sweltering day in the horse-farm and bluegrass country of central Kentucky, and many of my colleagues at the Sanders-Brown Center on Aging have gone home, while I've stayed on in the air-conditioned building to try to finish a grant proposal that is due next week.

After a couple of hours, I decide it's time for a break and head downstairs to Markesbery's laboratory. Cecil Runyons, his research assistant, is also working late. We're chatting when I spot a large UPS box on the black Formica counter near the door. Judging from the size of the box, I already know what is inside. Brains. These shipments make for an unusual office routine. *Any mail today? Not much. The usual junk mail . . . a couple of scientific journals. Oh, and a UPS box containing human brains.*

By now we have received several hundred brains, coming

from all seven Notre Dame provinces in the United States, but the arrival of these shipments has never become routine for me. I ask Cecil if it's okay to open the box to see how many new brains we have. Four. I lift the gallon-sized plastic tubs out of the box, one by one, and read the label taped to each lid.

Name: Sister Cecilia	Age at death: 97	Weight in grams: 1,040
Name: Sister Wilhelmina	Age at death: 94	Weight in grams: 1,070
Name: Sister Frances	Age at death: 92	Weight in grams: 920
Name: Sister Elizabeth	Age at death: 82	Weight in grams: 1,190

I'm both curious and cautious. I've never forgotten Dave Wekstein's lesson: "Remember, somebody died." I know that every brain comes to us at a cost. Sometimes a sister who is ailing will say to me—always cheerfully—"Dr. Snowdon, you'll be getting my brain soon." And I always reply, "Hang in there, Sister. We're in no hurry."

Now I lift one container to the light and see the outline of the brain resting in the cloudy yellow formalin solution. As I do, I recall visiting a room behind the chapel at the Elm Grove convent, where the sisters preserved their collection of relics—precious bits of bone or tissue that commemorate saints and martyrs. In cathedrals around the world, relics such as these are encased in ornate vessels and revered for their special powers. As unscientific as it sounds, I feel my own sort of reverence toward this brain; what I hold in my hand is sacred. Its weight reminds me of my responsibility as the director of the Nun Study. Each brain represents a rich, vibrant life, and each brain offers a unique legacy to those who probe its mysteries.

Before the Nun Study, I had never seen a human brain. Amazing as the organ is, with its winding mountains of gray and white matter, the sight at first spooked me a bit. As I learned more about the intricacies of brains and saw ever more of them, my initial discomfort gave way to wonder and awe. My teacher in all this has been Bill Markesbery. If my parents were ever afflicted with Alzheimer's disease, Bill is the neurologist I would choose to treat them. But as involved as he is with his patients, he's never lost his zest for research. His associates joke that he would take his microscope with him on vacation if his wife, Barbara, would let him.

Markesbery's lab has a special microscope with two eyepieces, so that he can sit side by side with colleagues to look at slices of brain tissue only eight to ten microns thick. (A human hair is about 100 microns.) I find it fascinating to sit at the second eyepiece as Bill guides me through the maze of the brain. Even as he examines its tissue millimeter by millimeter, pinpointing abnormalities and tracing the characteristic signs of Alzheimer's, the brain maintains some of its secrets. Most of the brains neatly fit our expectations, with little or no evidence of disease in a tack-sharp sister and abundant damage seen in a sister who had dementia. But sometimes Markesbery finds little evidence of Alzheimer's in a sister who had the classic symptoms of the disease. And sometimes brains from other sisters who appeared mentally intact when alive show extensive evidence of Alzheimer's. Illuminating the relationship between the symptoms of the disease—the progressive, devastating loss of function—and the damage to the brain that causes those symptoms is a central focus of the Nun Study.

—

Nearly one hundred years after Alois Alzheimer first described the disease, it still defies a simple diagnosis for clinicians and pathologists alike. Dementia simply means "out of one's mind" in Latin. The diagnosis is usually made if three types of symptoms are present: There must be impairments in short-term memory, in another area of cognition (such as language), and, finally, in social or daily functioning (such as dressing). Dementia has, to date, at least sixty known causes. It may result from infection by a bacterium (as in untreated syphilis), by a virus (as in AIDS), or by a newly discovered infectious agent called a prion (as in Creutzfeldt-Jakob disease or its variant, mad-cow disease). Nutritional and metabolic disorders such as vitamin B_{12} deficiencies and hypothyroidism can cause dementia, as can drug side effects, toxins, tumors, strokes, and serious head trauma. (Boxing has its own disease, dementia pugilistica.) Finally, it may result from degenerative diseases such as Huntington's or Parkinson's—or Alzheimer's.

As we now know, diseases impact different people differently—from cancer to diabetes, influenza to pneumonia, gout to asthma. A disease that quickly causes a severe illness in one person may take years or even decades to cause symptoms in another. Some people develop classic symptoms, while others hardly show any typical symptoms at all. What is common to most Alzheimer's patients is their slow downward course of mental, physical, and social deterioration.

In a textbook case of Alzheimer's, the symptoms begin subtly. The person starts having trouble remembering the names of people and objects, whether it rained that morning, and other simple details of day-to-day life. Of course, these sorts of short-term memory lapses are experienced by everyone from time to time. However, in Alzheimer's they increase in frequency and severity over time. A person with Alzheimer's may repeatedly make the same request or tell the same story over and over, as if she can't remember what happened just minutes before. Reasoning, planning, and organizing become more difficult; some people may have difficulty preparing a meal or walking to a place they have visited many times.

The point at which a family seeks help varies widely. Some may be alarmed when a retired accountant can no longer complete a tax return; for others, inability to balance a checkbook may be the turning point. Treatment is often delayed by ageism—the prejudice that failing capacities are normal for the elderly. Research has shown that the average person has symptoms for several years before a clinician diagnoses Alzheimer's.

The diagnosis itself is a delicate blend of experienced clinical judgment, examinations such as the ones the Nun Study uses, and tests to rule out other causes of dementia. The American Psychiatric Association and other groups have developed detailed guidelines to distinguish non-Alzheimer's dementia from possible or probable Alzheimer's. But there is no definitive test—no blood workup or even brain scan—that can provide absolute certainty in a living person.

As the disease progresses, language skills continue to decline. People have more and more trouble finding the right words to describe an object or an experience. Reading and writing become increasingly frustrating processes. Some may have trouble recognizing the faces of friends and family members, or even distinguishing the family pet from a household object. Not only may the date escape them, they may not accurately recall the season or even the year. Some of the most difficult symptoms are emotional: The person may experience mood swings, depression and withdrawal, delusions, paranoia, or aggressive behavior.

In addition to these problems, most Alzheimer's patients who live long enough gradually lose the ability to dress, bathe, toilet, and feed themselves, even though their muscles may still work perfectly. This is the breaking point for many families who have been caring for the patient at home. In the last stages, often eight to ten years after diagnosis, patients become bedridden and incontinent and cease communicating verbally. The official cause of death is often pneumonia, medical complications of a fall, or multiple organ failure.

In the case of Alzheimer's, it is not until after death—upon brain autopsy—that the diagnosis can be moved from probable to definite. Even here there is room for debate. Researchers agree that the two most common features of an Alzheimer's brain are the plaques and tangles that Alois Alzheimer first described. Almost a century later, scientists are still debating the most basic issues first raised by Dr. Alzheimer: Which of the two Alzheimer's lesions are more important in damaging and killing brain cells? How many plaques and tangles must be evident, and in which parts of the brain, before it is considered to be an "Alzheimer's brain"?

These are far from academic questions. In labs around the world, the race is on to answer them, because we believe they may contain the key to the root causes of the disease—and to its ultimate prevention and treatment.

Shortly after a brain arrives in Markesbery's lab, he sends it across the street to the University of Kentucky Hospital, where a magnetic resonance imaging (MRI) machine scans the organ to determine the precise contours, density, and volume of its internal structures. The brain then returns to the Center on Aging for a complete evaluation, both with the naked eye (the gross exam) and with the aid of a microscope (the micro exam).

Even a nonspecialist can immediately see one effect of the destruction caused by Alzheimer's. A healthy adult female brain usually weighs between 1,100 and 1,400 grams—approximately two-and-a-third to three pounds. The brains of most Alzheimer's patients are noticeably smaller; they often shrink below 1,000 grams, as the disease destroys brain tissue. The intricate, tightly packed ruts and grooves of the cerebral cortex, which forms the surface of the brain, are also changed. Now they appear as pronounced mountains and valleys, with gaping spaces between them.

Markesbery starts his gross exam by weighing the brain and rotating it in his latex-gloved hands, looking for abnormalities. Based on the height and depth of the surface mountains and valleys, he grades the degree of atrophy (loss or shrinkage) of brain tissue. He then places the brain on the tabletop, where his assistant, Cecil, photographs it from several angles. These digitized images are stored in the computer for later examination. Next, with a blade that resembles a bread knife, Markesbery cuts the brain into a dozen vertical half-inch slices. These cross sections are again photographed. Then, one by one, Markesbery visually inspects each slice, looking for abnormalities in the color, texture, and structure. Sometimes he can immediately see evidence of old head trauma, or arteries clogged by fatty deposits (called atherosclerotic plaques), or the discolored pits where small strokes have destroyed the tissue.

Now Markesbery prepares for his microscopic examination of the brain. First he delicately extracts sixteen samples, each about the size of a nickel, from several of the cross sections containing key regions of the brain. Over the next few weeks these are washed, chemically processed, and eventually embedded in small blocks of wax, which a special machine cuts into ultrathin shavings. A lab technician carefully places the slivers of tissue and paraffin on glass slides and then stains each sample with one of half a dozen dyes. The Bielschowsky silver stain, the dye that Dr. Alzheimer used in the early 1900s, is still used today to highlight the two primary lesions of the disease.

Under the microscope, the plaques make the tissue look dirty—like dark, soiled spots on a piece of cloth. They are formed from a protein called beta-amyloid, which usually exists in the brain in soluble form. However, in Alzheimer's, for reasons we still don't understand, the amyloid aggregates and forms these solid deposits we refer to as plaques.

The tangles of Alzheimer's appear as dark flames or tadpolelike shapes. They are made up of a protein called tau. In a healthy nerve cell, normal tau helps form ropelike structures called microtubules, which act as a sturdy skeleton. The microtubules are essential to how the nerve cell communicates with other neurons. They guide cell nutrients and chemical messages from the main cell body down the long tail (called the axon) that sends the messages on to other cells. However, in Alzheimer's disease, an abnormal form of tau accumulates, tangling the microtubules. The lines of communication are destroyed, and the cell is starved and immobilized. This crippled nerve cell then dies an early death.

The microscopic exam of the plaques and tangles requires the patience and focus for which Markesbery and his colleagues are famous. In each of the main thinking regions of the brain, the plaques and tangles are counted square millimeter by square millimeter, until an average is calculated. It is not just the overall number of plaques and tangles that is important for diagnosing Alzheimer's. The pathologist needs to know the average lesion count in key areas, and the pattern by which these lesions have invaded the brain.

In 1991 German researchers Heiko and Eva Braak published a study that showed how the location of tangles could be used to define six distinct stages of the disease. Stage 0 signifies the absence or rarity of tangles, and stages I through VI map the increasing number and spread of the tangles through the thinking regions of the brain.

In the course of their staging studies, for which they autopsied more than eight hundred brains, the Braaks and their colleagues also discovered that tangle-related lesions appear in people as young as twenty. And although the Braaks didn't have autopsy samples for people younger than twenty, they have proposed that Alzheimer's disease may be developing even in adolescents. They estimate that it may take fifty years or more for the Alzheimer's pathology to progress from stage I to stage V or VI, the most severe stages.

Based on the findings of the Braaks and other scientists, it is now believed that tangles first surface in the entorhinal cortex, a region located near the base of the skull that is important for memory. The tangles then move higher and deeper into the brain, invading the hippocampus and neighboring tissues. The hippocampus, which is named (in Greek) for the seahorse shape it takes in cross section, is also critical to learning and memory. One of its functions is to process and store new information so that we can recall it later.

Finally, the tangles reach the upper layer of the top of the brain, the neocortex. The neocortex is the brain's executive: Among other things, it orients us in time, orchestrates both the interpretation and expression of language, and sorts through the myriad visual, auditory, and olfactory stimuli from the environment. It ultimately decides—based on past learning and present circumstances—which of our impulses to allow and which to inhibit. It also permits our greatest intellectual achievements and the enormous range, subtlety, and flexibility of our social behavior.

The spread of the tangles from the entorhinal cortex (Braak stages I and II) to the hippocampus (stages III and IV) to the neocortex (stages V and VI) parallels, in part, the general pattern of the progressive loss of mental, physical, and social functioning that occurs in Alzheimer's patients.

This, of course, is a very rough sketch of an awesomely complex picture. Bill Markesbery constantly emphasizes how little we still know about the brain. We can't just peg a given function to a certain region, because the regions work in tandem. Learning takes place and memories are stored as a result of simultaneous processing and communication among the entorhinal cortex, the hippocampus, and the neocortex. As Alzheimer's pathology spreads from one of these areas to the next, memory and thinking are exponentially confounded.

Many neuroscientists believe that the brain devotes most of its resources to communication among the brain cells themselves—as if the brain were constantly talking to itself. Some call the brain a giant hologram. Others compare it to a huge network of computers, all engaged in parallel processing. Whichever image you choose, Alzheimer's increasingly shuts down the vital cross talk that makes us who we are.

———

One of the most striking features of the Nun Study is that Markesbery does his examinations "blind"—without knowing in advance the mental status of the sister whose brain is being studied. Pathologists normally like to know the patient's symptoms before interpreting the sometimes ambiguous findings present at autopsy. Jim Mortimer, however, somehow convinced Markesbery that a cloud might hang over his findings if he knew in advance how a sister had performed on our cognitive tests. In fact, a primary question the Nun Study tries to answer is how the pathology in the brain relates to the expression of the symptoms of Alzheimer's.

Only after Markesbery and his team complete their gross and microscopic examinations do we hold what is called a consensus conference, where we attempt to match his pathology findings with the results from our annual mental and physical testing of the sisters.

I attend every consensus conference, but a few stand out in my memory. One was the afternoon we met to discuss the findings for my dear friend Sister Maria, who had been so disabled at the end of her life that she did not recognize me. In addition to Markesbery, assembled in my office that day were Kathryn Riley, the study's neuropsychologist (and president of the local Alzheimer's Association chapter), and several other members of our research team. These conferences are well attended because Markesbery's report reveals so much about how the pathology of the brain relates to mental, physical, and social function. While most of this is old hat to Markesbery, even he has been surprised by findings that challenge some of our basic beliefs about Alzheimer's disease.

"Okay," Markesbery said, signaling that he was ready to begin the conference. He spread out in front of him the gross report and the computer forms documenting what he'd found.

"This is an eighty-two-year-old lady. The brain weighed one thousand one hundred and sixty grams." (This was well within normal range.) "There was marked atherosclerosis of the circle of Willis,"—the main bed of blood vessels that feed the brain. "There were four pinhead areas of darkened hemorrhage in the left parieto-occipital junction," which is located in the neocortex. But in Markesbery's judgment, neither the atherosclerosis nor the tiny hemorrhages were likely to have impaired her cognitive abilities.

"There's a mild degree of atrophy in the frontal lobe," he noted. (Again, this indicated some damage to the neocortex.) And then he reported the microscopic evidence, precisely ticking off the average number of plaques and tangles in different regions of the brain. Sister Maria had some but not an overwhelming number of plaques and tangles in her hippocampus and neocortex. On the Braak scale, he considered her only stage II.

It was now Kathy Riley's turn to review Sister Maria's scores on the three evaluations she took before her death. There was no question in Riley's mind that Sister Maria had the progressive loss of mental, physical, and social functioning characteristic of Alzheimer's disease.

Then we all looked at each other, completely baffled.

Clearly, Sister Maria's exams showed a classic Alzheimer's pattern. But the conventional wisdom at that time was that Alzheimer's symptoms emerged at Braak stages V or VI. Sister Maria was only a stage II. When we compared the number of tangles in her hippocampus to that found in other sisters analyzed earlier, she fell in the twenty-fifth percentile, meaning that 75 percent of the sisters had more lesions in this region.

As Markesbery sometimes says, "I used to know what Alzheimer's was." It is cases such as this that stretch our understanding of the connection between symptoms and brain pathology. Evidence from the Nun Study and other research is now starting to confirm that Sister Maria's case was not an anomaly and that Alzheimer's symptoms may indeed emerge as early as Braak stage II.

Everyone at the consensus conference was aware of the association between depression and Alzheimer's. We speculated that Sister Maria's long history of depression may have worked in tandem with her modest Alzheimer's pathology to bring on her symptoms. Since then, new findings have suggested a possible biological link between the two conditions. It is well established that the hippocampus atrophies, or shrinks, as Alzheimer's progresses. Recent research suggests that patients with chronic depression also have slight atrophy of the hippocampus. This could have been one of the things that tipped the scale for Sister Maria.

One case has little meaning by itself. But combined with the other data that the Nun Study is amassing, we have begun to illuminate the links between Braak staging and the observable symptoms of the disease. Of sisters in stages I or II, only 22 percent had evidence of dementia. For stages III and IV, that jumped to 43 percent. And by stages V and VI, 70 percent of the sisters had dementia.

As we remind ourselves when we are faced with a case such

as Sister Maria's, true understanding comes from combining the expected with the unexpected, from attempting to mesh what makes sense with what does not—and from remaining open to the facts, even when they challenge everything we thought we knew.

⟵

Sister Margaret's brain made perfect sense.

In the late 1990s Sister Margaret died at the age of ninety-one. By then we had closely evaluated her mental and physical function for six years. Sister Margaret had taught elementary school for more than fifty years, and when we first evaluated her, at age eighty-five, she could still easily care for herself, identify familiar objects, quickly name animals (eleven in sixty seconds), and draw geometric shapes of increasing complexity. Yet she had severe difficulty with the same Delayed Word Recall test that had so perplexed Sister Maria: Sister Margaret scored a zero. Although her strong performances in the other tests ruled out dementia, her failure to recall words she had learned five minutes earlier raised a red flag.

The next three batteries of tests we did—when she was eighty-seven, eighty-eight, and ninety years old—confirmed our concern. Sister Margaret had a stepwise, progressive decline in language and cognition, the classic pattern of Alzheimer's. She also steadily lost the ability to care for herself. By her last exam she scored a zero on every test. On her third and fourth exams we also asked for samples of her writing. Both times she only made a few ink marks on the page.

When Markesbery presented his pathology results at the consensus conference, they fit perfectly with the clinical report. Her brain weighed only 970 grams, below the 1,000-gram minimum standard for a healthy adult female brain. His notes from the gross examination showed moderate atrophy of the frontal lobe of the neocortex and some atherosclerosis in the arteries that fed her brain. However, given the cautiousness with which he approaches his work, he would not make a diagnosis based on these gross findings alone.

The microscopic findings were definitive. Sister Margaret had more tangles in her hippocampus than we had found in 90 percent of the other brains evaluated for the Nun Study—in the language of our project, she was in the ninetieth percentile. Her neocortex also had an abundance of tangles, placing her in the seventieth percentile, and it was riddled with plaques as well. Overall, Markesbery scored her as a stage V on the Braak scale.

We have come to see Alzheimer's as a continuum. Sister Margaret presents one extreme. The disease had devastated her brain, and it is a wonder that she did not develop more serious symptoms earlier. Had she died at age eighty-five, when we first examined her and she had problems only with short-term memory, no one but a pathologist would even have suggested that she had Alzheimer's. Sister Maria, in contrast, had modest pathological evidence of Alzheimer's disease but serious symptoms at eighty—years earlier than Sister Margaret. Does the difference lie in brain reserve, the ability of the brain to resist expressing the symptoms of the disease? Depression? Or some other factor altogether? These are questions to which we are still seeking answers.

—

Two other extraordinary cases stand out in my memory.

Sister Bernadette died of a massive heart attack in the mid-1990s at the age of eighty-five. When Markesbery and Riley convened our consensus conference a few months later, Markesbery, as usual, gave his pathology report first. Sister Bernadette's brain weight, 1,020 grams, sat at the border of normal. Looking at her brain with his naked eye, Markesbery found evidence of strokes, but he noted that these could have occurred at the time of the heart attack that killed her.

The microscopic analysis of her brain tissue, however, left little doubt that Alzheimer's disease had spread far and wide. Tangles cluttered her hippocampus and her neocortex, all the way up to the frontal lobe. Her neocortex had an abundance of plaques as well. Markesbery ranked her as a Braak stage VI, indicating the most severe presence of Alzheimer's pathology.

"I suppose you're now going to tell me that she was mentally intact," he joked as he finished his report. By then he had grown accustomed to the occasional disconnect between his pathology findings and Riley's cognitive records.

All eyes turned to Riley. "Yes," Riley said. "She was mentally intact." She had normal scores for each one of our mental and physical tests.

Riley then told us that Sister Bernadette, who had a master's degree, had taught elementary school for twenty-one years and high school for another seven. She had taken the Nun Study tests when she was eighty-one, eighty-three, and eighty-four years old. On each exam she scored high, showing no mental deterioration at all, not even a hint. In a particularly impressive videotaped exchange done with each exam, Sister Bernadette—without looking at a clock or a watch—stated the time within four minutes of the actual time. I recalled with sadness that on my friend Sister Maria's last exam, she could not tell whether it was morning or afternoon.

"Maybe this has something to do with it," one of the technicians offered. "Look at the initial MRI scan. It shows an unusual amount of gray matter." As it turned out, Sister Bernadette had more gray matter—formed by the cell bodies of neurons in the neocortex—than 90 percent of the other sisters we'd studied.

Sister Bernadette represented an extreme example: Despite

an abundance of plaques and tangles in her neocortex, the function of that brain region seemed to be incredibly preserved. It was as if her neocortex was resistant to destruction for some reason. Sister Bernadette appears to have been what we, and others, have come to call an "escapee." Death had intervened before her symptoms had time to surface.

The consensus conference for Sister Rose was memorable for another reason. Like Sister Bernadette, she had very high mental test scores until she died. (Her short-term memory test score was 8 out of 10, a level of performance enjoyed by only one out of four Nun Study participants.)

I knew Sister Rose as a quiet, thoughtful person—who, by the way, had lived to be one hundred years old. She had used her brain for a full century—she taught grade school for more than fifty years—without developing *any* clinical or pathological evidence of Alzheimer's disease. Her brain weighed a healthy 1,280 grams and showed no abnormalities on Markesbery's gross evaluation. Microscopic examinations revealed that she was a Braak stage 0, with only a couple of tangles in her entire brain. "An amazing brain," Markesbery proclaimed with obvious pleasure.

For all of us who hope to live a long time, this is extraordinarily good news, and it is supported by other research. Heiko Braak and his colleagues found that nearly 40 percent of the people in their study who died between the ages of ninety-six and one hundred ranked as stage I or stage 0, suggesting to them that some people may be relatively resistant to the development of Alzheimer's disease. If such resistant people do exist, then of course we want to know why, which once again raises the whole host of questions that the Nun Study explores. Was it their diets? Their genes? Their immune systems? Their education? Or something else in their life history or environment that we have still to discover?

Some people, such as Sister Margaret, fit our tidy definitions, with their clinical and pathological statuses dovetailing. The Nun Study's real eye-opening findings, however, are the ones that add to the evidence that Alzheimer's is not a yes/no disease. Rather, it is a process—one that evolves over decades and interacts with many other factors. We have shown dramatically how pathology alone often can mislead. Sister Bernadette had widespread damage and no symptoms, and our data now tell us that about a third of the sisters in stages V and VI have shared her "escapee" fate. And then there is Sister Maria, who had obvious symptoms and only modest damage. And finally there is Sister Rose, the centenarian who taught us what may indeed be the Nun Study's most amazing lesson: Alzheimer's disease is not an inevitable consequence of aging.

7

One with the Words

*Now I am wandering about in "Dove's Lane" waiting, yet only
three more weeks, to follow in the footprints of my Spouse,
bound to Him by the Holy Vows of Poverty, Chastity,
and Obedience.*

—Sister Emma

Another ride with a group of nuns stands out in my
memory. This time we're not crammed into the family
station wagon, but ensconced in the back of a black
stretch limousine. The three School Sisters of Notre Dame,
who came from the Milwaukee province, noticed the bottles
of champagne that had been put on ice for us, but no one was
interested. They were clearly feeling anxious on this short ride
from the Sheraton Hotel to Rockefeller Plaza. So was I. And
not because of the Manhattan morning madness.

Our trip to New York, including the swank hotel and the
limo ride, came courtesy of *Donahue*, the talk show that featured Phil Donahue, the Chicagoan with the thatch of white
hair who became famous for strolling through the studio audience, microphone in hand. People often said they could still
see the polite, smart Catholic-school boy in him. So it seemed

appropriate that on this day—September 15, 1994—we would be the guests on his show. Shortly after we arrived at the NBC studios and were ushered into the green room, we learned the provocative, if wildly overstated, title of our segment: "Did Some Old Milwaukee Nuns Discover the Answer to Alzheimer's?"

Earlier that summer, the Nun Study had had its first taste of fame. It began with a story in *Life* magazine that featured a dramatic, mystical photograph of one of Markesbery's technicians, Ela Patel, holding up a brain wreathed in a thin cloud of smoke. (The picture did not show the bowl of dry ice that provided the effect.) *Nightline*'s Ted Koppel followed, opening his show with a taped segment that featured the Mankato sisters doing aerobics while sitting in their chairs, Markesbery in his lab surrounded by brains in plastic tubs, and both Mortimer and me discussing the implications of the study. The *Donahue* show would take the Nun Study to an even wider audience, and it featured three participants who clearly demonstrated that age does not equal mental frailty: eighty-six-year-old Sister Dorothy Marie Zimmerman, a quiet and thoughtful former language professor and author; Sister Vincetta Vilker, a beautiful eighty-one-year-old retired high school teacher; and Sister Annina Hemczak, a jovial seventy-seven-year-old who had been a teacher and principal of elementary and high schools and still sometimes operated the convent's telephone switchboard.

Phil Donahue greeted us briefly in the green room, and then we were taken away to have our faces prepared for the lights and cameras. Sister Annina commented that she'd last worn makeup as a young girl before she'd entered the convent.

Suddenly, in a rush, we were onstage. Donahue opened with an overview of the Nun Study that included a video of some of the sisters at Elm Grove. Then he turned to the sisters, probing for explanations as to why their minds had fared so well. Sister Vincetta confirmed Donahue's suggestion that their "peaceful" lifestyles might be a factor. Sister Annina agreed with a comment from the audience about the importance of continuing to learn; she noted with pride that she had started taking piano lessons three years earlier, at age seventy-four. But Sister Dorothy won the most attention from Donahue, who, with his trademark flair, asked her questions that displayed her deep intelligence.

Sister Dorothy described a language laboratory that she had established and run for forty years at Mount Mary College, the School Sisters of Notre Dame school in Milwaukee. She then explained that she had also spent years translating from French the letters of St. Peter Fourier, whom she described as "something like the grandfather of our order." Sister Dorothy had written a biography of Fourier, who lived from 1565 to 1640 and started a congregation of sisters in France. When the School Sisters of Notre Dame were established in Bavaria in 1833, they based many of their own rules on those of Fourier's congregation. "The Bibliothèque Nationale in Paris sent me microfilms of his letters," noted Sister Dorothy. "These were handwritten. They had never been printed. It was very difficult."

"So you had to interpret script as well as the French, and then bring your own skills to presenting this in English," marveled Donahue.

"Not only that," Sister Dorothy added. "In the nineteenth century, France revised its spelling system."

Donahue wanted to wow the audience with Sister Dorothy's intellect in order to hammer in the notion that people who have developed their minds might have a reduced incidence of Alzheimer's.

He turned to me to make the point: "Are people with higher intelligence less likely to get Alzheimer's?" I groaned inwardly, and my friends later told me they could see me grimace on camera. This was not a road I wanted to go down on a talk show. I knew where it would lead: to much consternation and little clarity.

Donahue pressed on. "Is there any evidence that members of this religious order who did menial tasks—who did tasks that were not intellectually challenging—were more likely to contract Alzheimer's than those who were intellectually engaged?"

The word *menial* stung me. It brought back the hurt the home service sisters had felt when I first described our findings about education. Besides, the home service sisters I knew were devoted and skilled—they performed many tasks in the convent so that the other sisters could devote their energies to teaching.

Rather than answer directly, I began to describe our recent research. "When these women were in their twenties, just a few days before they took their vows, they all wrote autobiographies," I began. "We've discovered that those who had the richest vocabulary, the most complex sentences, the most ideas in their sentences—sixty years later, those were the sisters who got on *Donahue*." I gestured toward Sisters Dorothy, Annina, and Vincetta.

Luckily, we had to break for a commercial, and I saw the producer hand Donahue a handwritten sheet of paper. When the taping resumed, Donahue shifted his attention again to Sister Dorothy—I was relieved the spotlight was off me. Waving the paper in the air, he began, "The doctor has talked about your autobiographies. You wrote this in 1928, when you were twenty."

He quickly summarized the opening of Sister Dorothy's autobiography, which described how the idea of a religious vocation had grown in her. Following her first communion, she began to go to church every day. "Then you wrote this sentence," said Donahue. He read aloud in a measured cadence, pausing here and there for effect:

> *In these visits I prayed for martyrdom. I think these daily visits and my devotion to the Sacred Heart disposed the Heart of Jesus to regard my petition favorably, for we are told that religious life is a species of martyrdom.*

"Age twenty," said Donahue. "Well aren't you one with the words!"

After the taping, the sisters and I returned to the green room, where Donahue soon came by to say thank you. Having shed his suit and tie for blue jeans and tennis shoes, he walked around the room shaking each sister's hand. When he came to Sister Dorothy, she locked on to his hand.

"I have one more thing I want to tell you." She had been waiting all day to have this moment, and she was not about to let him go.

"What's that, Sister?"

"I want to tell you a story about the Pope."

Donahue gave a slight smile.

"When I had an audience with the Pope in Rome, I told him I was a School Sister of Notre Dame. Do you know what he said?"

"No, Sister. What was it?"

"The Pope said to me, 'Congratulations on your football team.' "

Of course, the School Sisters of Notre Dame have nothing to do with the University of Notre Dame—or their football team. Donahue's smile turned into a wide grin.

Sister Dorothy pulled the talk show host closer. In a mock-serious stage whisper she said, "He's lucky I didn't tackle him for saying that!"

Yes, Sister Dorothy was "one with the words." And two years

later our careful study of autobiographies from ninety-three Milwaukee sisters would lead to the Nun Study's first publication in a high-profile medical journal. This meant far more to us than the attention from *Donahue, Nightline,* and *Life.*

—

Almost as soon as I discovered the autobiographies in the archives at Mankato, Jim Mortimer and I realized that they were fossils of a sort—miraculously preserved fragments of the past that might help us better understand the sisters' mental function early in life. But Jim and I had few concrete ideas how these fragments might fit together into a recognizable and meaningful form. Two new colleagues showed us where to dig and how to evaluate what we found.

I hired Lydia Greiner, a nurse who had graduate training in physical and medical anthropology, soon after I moved to Lexington. Greiner had a talent for seeing patterns that might have been missed by a less acute eye. Some of the autobiographies, which typically ran one or two pages, were typed, while others were handwritten. I thought nothing of the distinction, but Greiner decided right away that we could not use the typed ones. We had no way of verifying their authenticity, she pointed out: Someone other than the author might have done the typing, changing words or even entire thoughts and thus compromising the authenticity of the prose. Similarly, Greiner found several instances in which one scribe appeared to have handwritten more than one autobiography. We discarded these samples from our analysis, too.

Greiner focused on the Milwaukee convent and determined that ninety-three autobiographies had been handwritten in the first person by sisters who took their vows between 1931 and 1939. (The earlier years yielded only a few handwritten autobiographies, so we excluded them.) Greiner then separated these sisters into one group that had clinical symptoms of Alzheimer's and another that did not, our healthy controls. Next we had to determine how to analyze the differences between these two groups. This proved more difficult than we had imagined.

Jim Mortimer and I suspected that a rich vocabulary in early life would identify those sisters with highly developed cognitive skills and well-wired brains. Later in life such verbally adept sisters might have more resistance to Alzheimer's disease. Mortimer and I settled on two measures of vocabulary and set about the tedious labor of testing our hypothesis.

First we assessed the use of monosyllabic and multisyllabic words. I created a database of all the words used in the Milwaukee autobiographies, and then Greiner and I painstakingly counted the number of syllables in each word. Our subsequent computer analysis tended to confirm that the healthy controls were more apt to use multisyllabic words, such as *particularly, privileged,* and *quarantined.* In contrast, the sisters who later developed Alzheimer's more frequently used monosyllabic words, such as *girls, boys,* and *sick.*

Our second gauge of vocabulary measured the frequency of rarely used words in the autobiographies. To do this, we turned to a database of ten thousand words that had been prepared in 1921 by psychologist Edward Thorndike, a Columbia University professor and researcher. Thorndike had surveyed four million words from forty-one sources that included the Bible, English-language classics, textbooks, the U.S. Constitution, and daily newspapers to determine how often each of the ten thousand words were used in 1921, the time when our study participants were children or young adults.

This second approach to vocabulary was even more productive than the first. Common multisyllabic words, such as *religious,* were used by both the sisters who later developed Alzheimer's and the healthy controls. But the controls also used words, such as *grandeur,* that Professor Thorndike had only rarely encountered in the literature of the early part of the twentieth century. This suggested that the healthy sisters had a richer vocabulary in early life and may have read a more diverse selection of literature as children.

These data intrigued us, but they raised as many questions as they seemed to answer. Was it the words the sisters used or the combinations of words that best revealed their cognitive skills? Maybe it was the complexity of the sentences that we should analyze. Should we be counting clauses? Verbs? Conjunctions? A grant application to study these questions led us to someone who could guide us through this maze.

The National Institute on Aging, which funds most of our work, supports academic investigators whose grant proposals fare the best when reviewed by scientists working in the same field. During this peer-review process, the researchers who evaluated our proposal suggested that we needed a language expert to help us determine whether the autobiographies truly held valuable information about our subjects' cognitive or linguistic abilities or whether they simply offered intriguing glimpses into the past. The grant reviewers even went so far as to suggest a specific researcher: Dr. Susan Kemper, a psycholinguist with specialized knowledge about the impact of aging on language skills.

When I read Kemper's publications, I realized that there were an astonishing number of tools to analyze language that we had never considered. In addition to vocabulary, she and her associates assessed such odd-sounding parameters as morphemes, left- and right-branching sentences, embedded clauses, verb phrase infinitive complexes, conceptual propositions, lexical repetition, and anaphora. After I phoned her and described the project, she agreed to look at a few autobiographies. A few weeks later we had an enthusiastic new collaborator.

Smart scientists, like experienced mechanics or carpenters, not only have amassed many tools, but also have a knack for selecting the best tools for the job at hand. Kemper suggested that the most powerful way to quantitatively gauge linguistic ability in these autobiographies was to measure idea density and, separately, grammatical complexity. Kemper defined idea density as the number of propositions (individual ideas) expressed per ten words. Grammatical complexity classified sentences on a scale that ranges from 0 (a simple one-clause sentence) to 7 (complex sentences with many forms of embedding—grammatical units nested within larger units—and subordination).

Kemper explained to me that idea density reflects language processing ability, which in turn is associated with a person's level of education, general knowledge, vocabulary, and reading comprehension. Grammatical complexity, on the other hand, is associated with working memory capacity. In order to write a complex sentence, Kemper pointed out, you have to keep many elements in play, juggling them until they are all properly coordinated. There's always a risk of losing your train of thought before you reach the end of the sentence.

I asked her how a writer such as Ernest Hemingway, who was famous for fashioning simple sentences, might rank in this type of analysis. "I have never claimed that complex sentences or idea-dense sentences make for good literature," said Kemper. But they did, as it turned out, offer us an extraordinary tool in our pursuit of the mysteries of Alzheimer's disease.

━

Kemper and her associates would analyze the autobiographies blind, with no knowledge of the sisters' current mental or physical condition.

In some cases, striking differences were apparent from the very first sentence.

I was born in Eau Claire, Wis., on May 24, 1913 and was baptized in St. James Church.

—Sister Helen

It was about a half hour before midnight between February twenty-eighth and twenty-ninth of the leap year nineteen-hundred-twelve when I began to live and to die as the third child of my mother, whose maiden name is Hilda Hoffman, and my father, Otto Schmitt.

—Sister Emma

When we evaluated all ninety-three autobiographies from nuns who were novices in Milwaukee province between 1931 and 1939, Sister Helen had the lowest scores for idea density and grammatical complexity. Sister Emma had the highest.

My father, Mr. L. M. Hallacher, was born in the city of Ross, County Cork, Ireland, and is now a sheet metal worker in Eau Claire.

—Sister Helen

My father is an all around man of trades, but his principal occupation is carpentry which trade he had already begun before his marriage with my mother.

—Sister Emma

You do not have to be a linguist to notice the differences in the way that these two sisters describe their lives. As a colleague once pointed out to me, it was as though one was a monophonic recording and the other was in high fidelity. For an even more dramatic example, consider the references they make to their siblings.

There are ten children in the family six boys and four girls. Two of the boys are dead.

—Sister Helen

Already two, a brother and a sister, had begun the family which would gradually reach the number of eight. . . . When I was in the fourth grade death visited our family taking one to whom I was very particularly attached, my little brother, Karl, who was but a year and a half old. He was called to his "Home" after three weeks of very much suffering on Good Friday early in the morning. The pastor was willing to have the funeral services conducted before Easter, but I was hoping and praying that my parents would not consent, for I thought since he died on Good Friday he might be in our midst, living, on Easter Sunday. The services were held on Monday morning which I was privileged to attend since we were quarantined.

—Sister Emma

Or consider how they end their autobiographies.

I prefer teaching music to any other profession.

—Sister Helen

Now I am wandering about in "Dove's Lane" waiting, yet only three more weeks, to follow in the footprints of my Spouse, bound to Him by the Holy Vows of Poverty, Chastity, and Obedience.

—Sister Emma

When we opened our records and discovered who had written which autobiography, we discovered that the sisters' fates differed as much as their writing styles. The sisters in our sample had started out on the same educational footing. Both Sisters Helen and Emma had twelve years of education at the time they wrote their autobiographies. Both went on to receive their bachelor's degrees. Sister Helen also earned an M.A. When they were first assessed for the Nun Study in 1992, Sister Emma had a score of 30 on the Mini-Mental State Exam, the highest possible score for this test of overall cognitive function. Sister Helen, however, scored a 0. A year later Sister Helen died, at age eighty, and Markesbery's autopsy confirmed the diagnosis of Alzheimer's disease. Sister Emma was still alive and fully mentally intact.

Despite the obvious contrast between these two writing samples, it did not take on any real scientific meaning until Susan Kemper had quantified all ninety-three autobiographies and we compared those results to the scores on the battery of cognitive tests that the sisters had taken every year. What we found astonished us.

The level of idea density in the autobiographies was strongly associated with the scores from our cognitive tests. Grammatical complexity was also associated with the test scores, but the relationship was weaker. This led us to focus our analysis on idea density.

We classified sisters as having low idea density if their scores fell in the bottom third of the group. The remainder of the group—the top two-thirds—were classified as having high idea density. For each cognitive test, the prevalence of impairment was dramatically higher in those with low idea density. For example, 35 percent of those with low idea density had scores on the Mini-Mental State Exam that suggested mental impairment (scores of less than 24 out of a possible 30). In contrast, only 2 percent of those with high idea density had scores this low.

On average, these sisters were twenty-two years old when they wrote their autobiographies and eighty when we assessed their mental function. Somehow, a one-page writing sample could, fifty-eight years after pen was put to paper, strongly predict who would have cognitive problems. We ruled out the possibility that this finding might have reflected the level of education or occupation in one group versus another: Fully eighty-five of the ninety-three sisters whose autobiographies we studied were college-educated and worked as teachers.

Jim Mortimer had hypothesized that intellectual stimulation throughout adulthood might be the key to keeping aging brains sharp and preventing Alzheimer's—an expansion of his idea of brain reserve. Here, however, this was clearly not a factor. "To me it was the most bizarre finding on earth," he later told *New York Times* reporter Gina Kolata. This study convinced him that Alzheimer's disease might well reflect a lifelong process, one that progressed very slowly and caused symptoms only when a certain level of damage was reached.

Our growing bank of brains allowed us to take this inquiry to the next level—confirmation in the laboratory. At the time of this analysis in 1995, fourteen of the ninety-three sisters—including Sister Helen—had died. Based on the count and location of tangles in their brains, Bill Markesbery concluded that five of the sisters had pathologically-confirmed Alzheimer's disease. Sister Helen had such extensive tangles in both her hippocampus and her neocortex that Markesbery rated her a Braak stage VI, indicating the most severe form of Alzheimer's. All five of the sisters with Alzheimer's had low idea density. The other nine autopsied brains that appeared healthy all belonged to sisters who had high idea density.

These results stunned us—but we did not completely trust them because we had so few brains to analyze. So we searched for handwritten autobiographies from other convents and uncovered eleven more from sisters whom Markesbery had autopsied. When they were added to our original sample, we had a total of twenty-five autobiographies from our autopsy pool, ten of whom had confirmed Alzheimer's. An amazing 90 percent of the women with Alzheimer's disease had low idea density in their autobiographies, as compared to only 13 percent of the healthy sisters.

This was a huge difference, and it suggested that within 85 to 90 percent accuracy, we could predict who would get Alzheimer's disease *about sixty years later* and who would not—simply by evaluating their autobiographies. Several years after this first study, after seventy-four sisters with early-life autobiographies had been autopsied, the power of idea density in predicting Alzheimer's disease in late life was about 80 percent—still an incredible level of accuracy.

I do not know why low idea density early in life predicts so strongly who will develop Alzheimer's. Conversely, I can only speculate about why high idea density seems to protect people such as Sister Emma. One potential explanation is that low idea density early in life indicates that the brain is already compromised in some way. This is corroborated by the Braaks' work on the staging of Alzheimer's disease pathology in the brain: Based on autopsies of the brains of 887 people who ranged in age from 20 to 104, the Braaks and their colleagues concluded that the tangle pathology of Alzheimer's is present in some twenty-year-olds and that the tangles develop over approximately fifty years.

In the end, we faced a chicken-and-egg dilemma. Did neuropathological changes early in life compromise a person's linguistic ability? Or did the low linguistic ability somehow speed up the development of plaques and tangles in mid- and later life?

In 1995 we submitted a paper to the *Journal of the American Medical Association* that described these findings—and these perplexing questions. While I was at lunch one day, a secretary gave Lydia Greiner the reply from the journal's editors. When I returned, I found a fantastic gift waiting for me on my desk: the open acceptance letter taped to a bottle of champagne.

—

Since I am 74 years old and getting older, I have often wondered what miracle has spared me from Alzheimer's disease. Now it turns out that simple, direct exposition, unornamented with lush adjectives and adverbs, puts one at high risk for Alzheimer's.

Let me tell you, I have never written a simple declarative sentence in my life. My writing style is complex, prolix, obfuscatory. It is as unfathomable as that of a doctoral candidate in sociology, or maybe even a psycholinguist's—if that is possible.

I am trying to hold my prose on a tight leash right now, but believe me, eschewing the tortured phrase is hard. Even as I write this, I feel myself getting more and more "idea dense"—so idea dense you couldn't separate one of my thoughts from another with a blow torch. I may live to be 150 before Alzheimer's gets me.

—Gordon Carlson, letter to the editor, *The New York Times*, February 24, 1996

When our paper appeared in the February 21, 1996, issue of the prestigious *Journal of the American Medical Association*, it attracted intense media coverage—and some intense scrutiny from both the public and our colleagues. The journal itself subsequently ran two critical letters to the editor. One suggested that we had made "a potentially important omission": the emotional content of the autobiographies. Perhaps, this writer suggested, emotionally expressive people fare better.

Actually, this was one of the first hypotheses that Lydia Greiner and I had come up with. The low-idea-density writers tended to be what we called "listers," in contrast to the more "emotional," "sensuous" high-density writers. However, additional analysis had revealed no relationship between emotional expression and cognitive function. Still, the stylistic difference was so striking that we were determined to return to it in a later study.

The second critic of our linguistic findings correctly noted that the psycholinguistic measures we used originally had been designed for another purpose: to assess how difficult a text was to read or understand. This writer asserted that the ability to comprehend difficult texts may well reflect high linguistic ability, but the ability to write them, he concluded, "reflects just the opposite." This complaint, similar to the witty letter to the editor of the *New York Times,* missed an important distinction. As we wrote in our reply, there was nothing "wrong" with either the high- or low-density sentences in our study. Both kinds of writers were grammatical, expressed clear ideas, and developed them in a cogent way. The sentences with high idea density are not difficult to understand. Many of them are vivid, almost poetic, in the way they link together complex ideas and events.

Finally we come back to the question I ducked on *Donahue* and which remains one of the most frequently asked questions about our work: How does intelligence relate to the differences we observed, and what do we know about the relationship between IQ and Alzheimer's? To begin with, we do not have standard measures of intelligence on the sisters during their young adult years; IQ testing did not begin in earnest until World War II. The convent records do, however, contain an indirect measure of intellectual performance: high school grades. Surprisingly, idea density was not related to the sisters' grades in subjects such as English, Latin, geometry, or algebra. This argues that verbal and analytic intelligence may not be reflected in idea density. Rather, idea density may signify other

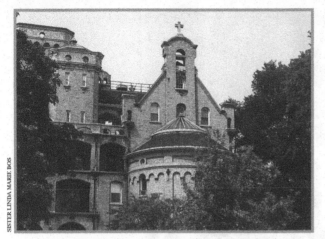

The convent of the School Sisters of Notre Dame in Elm Grove, Wisconsin, was established in 1859. The Nun Study enrolled 678 sisters from seven Notre Dame provinces in the United States.

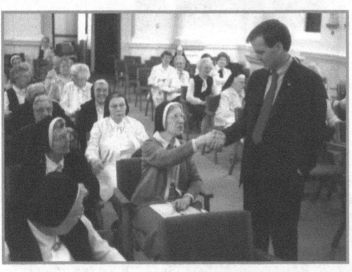

Asking the sisters to donate their brains to the Nun Study was one of the most difficult things I've ever done. Sister Loretta Semposki, with whom I'm shaking hands, was one of the first to sign on.

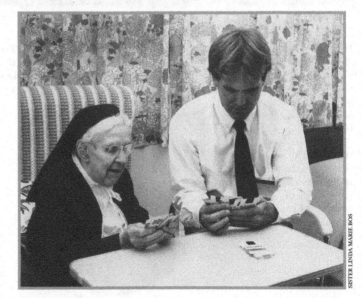

Many of the sisters, like Sister Columbine Kumba, have become part of my extended family.

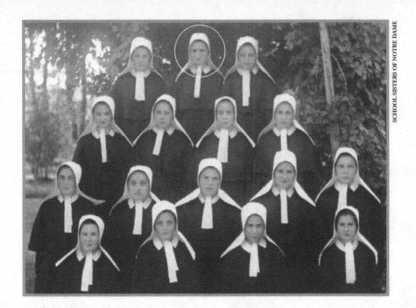

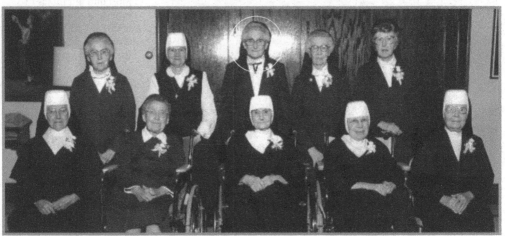

TOP: Following the sisters through their lifetimes is an integral feature of the Nun Study. Sister Nicolette Welter, *circled,* is shown here at age 18 with her class of postulants in 1925.

MIDDLE: The same class in 1987, on the 60th anniversary of their vows. Sister Nicolette, age 80, is again in the center. Mortality has already taken its toll.

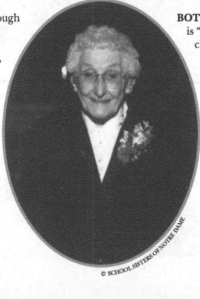

BOTTOM: Sister Nicolette, at age 90, is "the last nun standing" in her class. Since the sisters have very similar lifestyles, the Nun Study can focus on the key differences that enable some to enjoy robust health into old age.

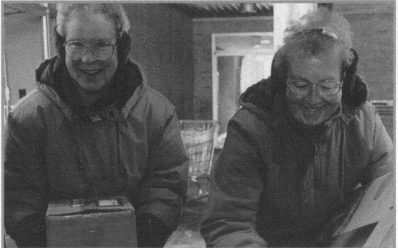

Sisters Marlene Manney, *left*, and Gabriel Mary Spaeth travel throughout the United States performing yearly evaluations on each Nun Study participant. Here they load their boxes of special equipment into the back of their van.

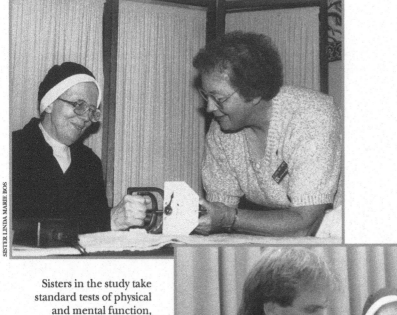

Sisters in the study take standard tests of physical and mental function, like this test of handgrip strength administered by Sister Gabriel Mary Spaeth. After the assessment each sister receives a computerized report of her results.

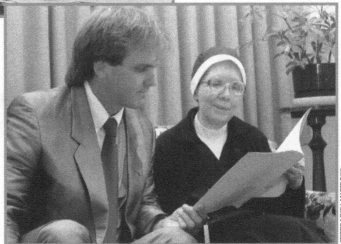

When I met Sister Dorothy Zimmerman, *center*, for the first time, this former language professor was celebrating her 86th birthday with a closely contested game of Scrabble. As the Nun Study reveals, verbal skills measured early in life predict later brain health with startling accuracy.

The Nun Study also draws on a wealth of records meticulously collected in the convent archives. Sister Genevieve Kunkel's autobiography, written nearly 70 years ago, contributed to one of our most surprising conclusions.

"Sister Sisters" Clarissa Gores, *left*, and Liguori Gores. Eighteen percent of the participants in the study have a sibling who is also a School Sister of Notre Dame. Being able to study genetically related sisters adds to the wealth of our data.

Sister Dolores Rauch left Germany for America after the Nazis took power. At age 67 she fulfilled her lifelong ambition to be a missionary in Africa, pioneering a successful reforestation project in Kenya. Since returning to the United States at age 80, she has continued to lecture and write about her missionary work.

© JUDY GRIESEDIECK

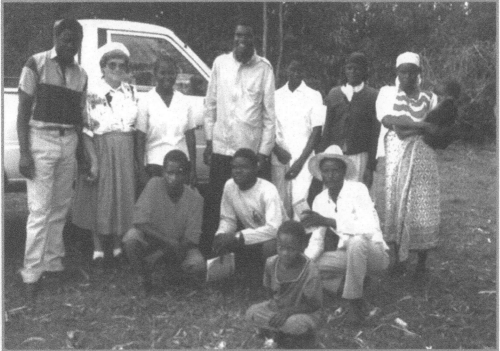

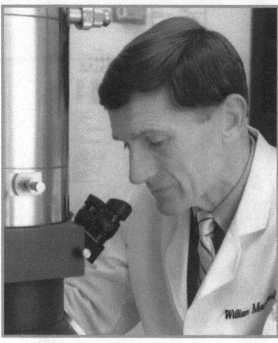

Neuropathologist Dr. William Markesbery performs his microscopic examinations of brain tissue "blind"— without knowing a sister's health status before her death. Astonishingly, the Nun Study has found that some sisters retain their mental acuity despite having extensive brain damage from Alzheimer's.

Slides of brain tissue are stained with dyes to highlight the spread of Alzheimer's throughout the brain.

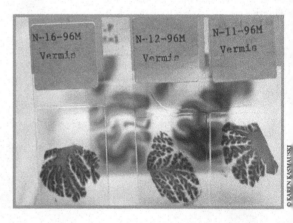

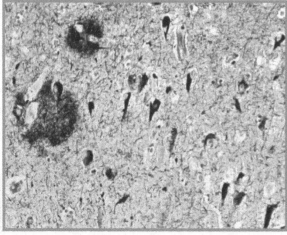

This microscopic image shows the characteristic lesions of Alzheimer's disease: the dark blob-like plaques and the tadpole-like tangles.

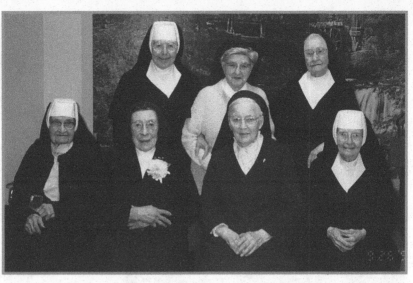

"The Magnificent Seven"—In 1995, the Mankato convent feted seven sisters who were over 100 years old. *Back row:* Sisters Marcella Zachman, Esther Boor, Borgia Leuther. *Front row:* Sisters Verena Koppy, Augustine Peterburs, Mary Clemens Slater, Matthia Gores.

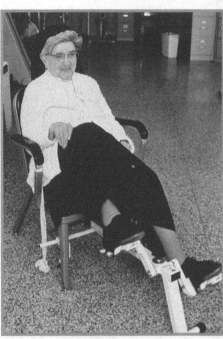

In December 2000 Sister Esther Boor celebrated her 106th birthday, making her the longest-lived School Sister of Notre Dame—and one of five Nun Study participants who have lived in three centuries.

Until her death less than one month before her 105th birthday, Sister Matthia Gores knitted a pair of mittens every day for the poor and prayed every evening for the 4,378 students she had taught over the years.

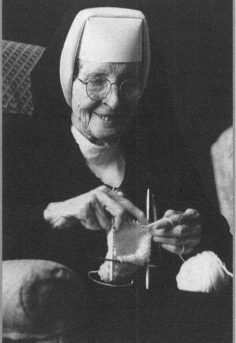

Centenarian
Sister Borgia Leuther.

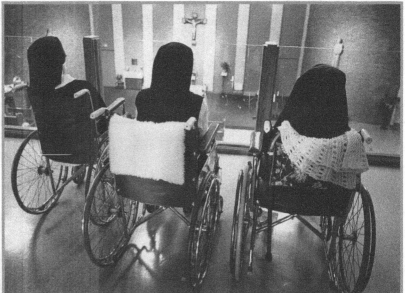

© JUDY GRIESEDIECK

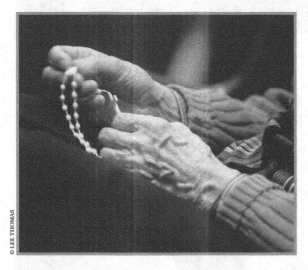

© LEE THOMAS

Prayer and worship are at
the core of the sisters' lives
at every age and stage of
health. While we cannot
directly measure intangi-
bles such as faith and social
support, the Nun Study
would be incomplete
without acknowledging
their powerful influence.

© LEE THOMAS

properties of the brain, such as those related to perception, encoding, and memory retrieval. At this point we simply do not know for sure.

—

The personal impact of this Nun Study data came home to me one afternoon in Bill Markesbery's office as Susan Kemper and I laid out our findings for him. Unexpectedly, Bill didn't ask us technical questions about our statistical and linguistic methods. He looked directly at Susan and said, "What does this mean for our children?"

The question caught me off guard. But when I saw the look on his face, I realized that he was speaking as a father, not a scientist. Bill has three grown daughters, and it was clear he wanted to know whether he and his wife, Barbara, had done the right things as parents.

"Read to them," Susan answered. "It's that simple. It's the most important thing a parent can do with their children."

Susan explained that idea density depends on at least two important learned skills: vocabulary and reading comprehension. "And the best way to increase vocabulary and reading comprehension is by starting early in life, by reading to your children," Susan declared.

I could see the relief spread over Bill's face. "Barbara and I read to our kids every night," he said proudly.

We now know that the brain is capable of changing and growing throughout life, but there is no question that most of its growth comes during our earliest years. Infants' and young children's brains grow exponentially after birth. Before sexual maturity, the brain is sculpted and innumerable connections between nerve cells are formed. This development is powerfully influenced by experience, so there *is* something we can do to increase and direct the brain's capacity.

In the years since our study came out, I have been asked Markesbery's question many times. Parents ask me if they should play Mozart to their babies, or buy them expensive teaching toys, or prohibit television, or get them started early on the computer. I give them the same simple answer Susan Kemper gave to Markesbery: "Read to your children."

My listeners nod with satisfaction, as if I had confirmed what they knew all along.

—

About a year after the linguistics study was published, I visited Sister Dorothy Zimmerman at the Marian Catholic nursing home. At the time of the *Donahue* taping, her bad knees had occasionally forced her to use a wheelchair; now she could not move without one. I stood outside the open door of Sister Dorothy's room for a few moments and watched her, unnoticed—at least by her. I was taken aback by the physical change in her appearance, and one of the nurses walking by must have seen the serious expression on my face. "Watch out for this one," she told me. "She may be in a wheelchair, but the wheels are still spinning fast in that head."

The *Donahue* experience had created a strong bond between Sister Dorothy and me, and when I entered her room, her face lit up. She sat near the window, a white afghan covering her legs. A folded section of a newspaper was resting in her lap.

"Reading the paper?" I asked.

"Oh, read it this morning. Now I'm just doing my puzzle." She opened the fold of the *New York Times* and showed me a crossword puzzle nearly completed in black ink. "It keeps me out of mischief," said this former language professor.

"Have you always been good with words?" I asked.

"Oh, yes."

"Why do you think you have that gift?"

"My childhood," she said. "You see, I grew up in Indiana, but my family has German and French roots. Every year my parents would always talk to each other in German about our Christmas presents so that we kids wouldn't understand. When I was five I taught myself the language so I would know what I was getting."

"You taught yourself German at age five?"

"Rudimentary German, mind you. For beginners. But not bad for a five-year-old," she said. "And all because I wanted to find out about my Christmas presents."

Sister Dorothy died on November 3, 1997, at the age of eighty-nine. The cause of death was heart disease. She had never shown any decline in any of our mental exams, and the nurses told me that she remained alert up until the day of her death. A brain autopsy revealed that she had a very small number of tangles in her hippocampus, but none in her neocortex. I was glad to know that Sister Dorothy's way with words—and the pleasure she took from them—had remained with her until the end.

8

Family Ties

Do you know what my worst fear was? That I was going to forget Jesus. I finally realized that I may not remember Him, but He will remember me.

—Sister Laura

Sister Louise caught up with me one morning after breakfast at one of the convents and asked if she could speak with me privately for a few minutes. We had become acquainted in the early days of the Nun Study, and her birthdays since—she was then ninety—had not diminished either her firm step or her sharp mind. We found an empty parlor and relaxed into a pair of broken-in, overstuffed chairs. Sister Louise leaned in close to me.

"Dr. Snowdon, I'm concerned about my sister Ann," she began. Sister Ann was Sister Louise's younger biological sister, and both had taken their vows in the same convent decades before. Fully 18 percent of the participants in the Nun Study have a sibling who is also a School Sister of Notre Dame, and from the outset I knew that they might provide unique information about the genetics of Alzheimer's disease. What never occurred to me until that morning is that they also would confront us with vexing ethical dilemmas.

Sister Louise was a few years older than Sister Ann, but she was still living in the retirement wing of the convent, while Sister Ann had moved to the assisted-living center after a series of small strokes had put her into a wheelchair. I knew that Sister Louise visited her sister several times a day. "Her doctor told me last year that she was slipping, but she'd been ailing off and on all winter, and I thought she'd come out of it," she explained. "But now sometimes when I see her in the afternoon, she doesn't seem to remember that I visited her that same morning. Still, when we're talking about our childhood—about something our father or mother did seventy-five years ago—she can recall the tiniest details. Do you think she could have Alzheimer's?"

I was touched—and a bit uncomfortable—that Sister Louise had come to me with this question. She was right to be concerned: Loss of short-term memory is *the* hallmark of Alzheimer's disease. But I also knew that Sister Ann had already been diagnosed with Alzheimer's after a thorough medical and neurological workup. I wondered if Sister Ann's doctor had softened the news somewhat in his conversations with Sister Louise, or if she simply hadn't been ready to accept it.

Now, however, she was bringing up the topic herself, and I thought that hedging on my part would only increase her anxiety. I had my laptop computer with me, which contains vast amounts of information about each sister in our study, including the results of a series of mental exams. "Give me one minute," I said to Sister Louise, thinking that showing her our data might provide a somewhat neutral way of telling the truth.

Sister Ann's mental exams indeed showed a steady decline over the last five years. (Sister Louise's own scores were considerably higher than Sister Ann's—well within normal range.) "And here's her DNA test," I said. "She has one copy of the APOE-4 gene on chromosome 19." Sister Louise looked me straight in the eye as I gave her a primer on the genetics of Alzheimer's disease.

As I outlined to Sister Louise, the DNA inside the human body contains tens of thousands of genes. As of 2001, the best estimate is around 30 thousand. Each of these genes, in turn, holds the code that tells the body to make a specific protein. Errors in a gene often lead to an improperly formed protein, which can lead to disease. Until 1992, hardly any Alzheimer's researchers had heard of apolipoprotein E, a protein that resides in the blood and tissue and helps the body shuttle cholesterol and other fats from place to place. That year, however, a team of researchers at Duke University Medical Center discovered that people who had a particular type of apolipoprotein E had much higher rates of Alzheimer's disease. Specifically, the proteins of apolipoprotein E occur in three forms—designated 2, 3, and 4—each of which is coded for by a variant of the "APOE" gene. People who inherit a copy of the APOE-4 variant from one parent, the Duke group reported, have nearly three times the normal risk of developing Alzheimer's disease. The risk for those who inherit the gene from both parents is about eight times higher than for someone who has no APOE-4 genes.

Sister Louise followed intently as I explained that a single APOE-4 gene did not necessarily mean that someone would develop Alzheimer's; rather, it suggested an increased susceptibility to the disease. However, combined with Sister Ann's test scores, the presence of the gene strengthened the likelihood that she was indeed suffering from Alzheimer's.

I have a Ph.D., not an M.D., and I make a point of never giving medical advice. But I also feel an obligation to share the latest medical information. I suggested to Sister Louise that she speak with Sister Ann's doctor about an Alzheimer's drug that was relatively new at that time: donepezil, also called by its brand name, Aricept. I warned her, however, not to expect too much from it—it could provide short-term help at best.

Aricept slows down the degradation of acetylcholine, a critical chemical that some nerve cells use to communicate with each other—and which Alzheimer's depletes. Even in the best cases, however, the drug only modestly slows the decline in cognitive function. It does not have any effect on the development of plaques or tangles or the destruction of tissue that leads to brain atrophy. Like similar drugs that have since become available, Aricept might be said to shore up the riverbank, but it still can't stop the flood.

"The real hope is that as we learn more about the genetics of Alzheimer's, it will become possible to develop drugs that get at the cause of the disease, not just its symptoms," I said. "And we have a lot to learn from you. You and Sister Ann are helping to combat Alzheimer's by participating in the Nun Study.

"Right now, your visits are probably the most important thing you can do for Sister Ann," I went on. "Discussing current events or recalling what you did when you were young may help reinforce her memory. You could read aloud, too, or sing songs together, or play cards or do some puzzles, if she enjoys those activities. Both the stimulation and the emotional support count for a lot." I added that discovering activities that Alzheimer's patients can actively participate in—at whatever level—helps them maintain enjoyment, pride, and dignity in their lives.

I was pretty sure that Sister Louise was already doing these things. I have always been moved by the amount of tender care and love the active sisters give to those who are failing, whether or not they are family members. But I wanted to reassure her that her love and attention could truly help her sister.

"We've also learned that Alzheimer's patients need plenty of time to respond," I said. "Some people forget to slow down their speech, or they start quizzing the patient with questions like 'You remember me, don't you?' I can't imagine you'd do that, but you might want to pass along the tip to Sister Ann's friends, who may be uncertain how to act around her."

Sister Louise thanked me, and we said our goodbyes. I hoped that what I'd said had eased her mind. It was not until the next morning that doubt set in—part of our conversation might have done just the opposite.

I had never before revealed the APOE-4 status of a Nun Study participant—and in the light of a new day, I vowed never to do so again without a compelling medical reason. By telling Sister Louise her sister's cognitive and genetic status, I had un-wittingly introduced the idea that she, too, might carry the gene. As it turned out, Sister Louise had not inherited it. But now if I went to her with that information, she might logically ask about her brother and her much-loved nieces and nephews. I did not want to cause further anxiety or become embroiled in a discussion about whether they should be tested.

As an epidemiologist, I see risk in mathematical terms: It is a way to gauge possibilities versus probabilities. But my work has taught me that nonscientists often view the concept of risk much differently. When people learn that they have a higher risk for a disease, it sometimes leads them to conclude that the illness either already has struck or soon will. And to live in fear of a disease that you do not have—and may never develop—exacts a high price.

—

Sister Laura impressed upon me just how costly the label of Alzheimer's disease can be.

In the early 1980s Sister Laura had been living in a small convent near the school where she taught. As she told me the story a decade later, her problems began when she was under a good deal of pressure at school. She found herself in a deepening depression—unable to sleep, unable to concentrate, and haunted by a sense that nothing and no one depended on her. She saw a doctor, who prescribed several of the medications available at the time, but they failed to provide any relief.

The doctor then asked her to take a brain CAT scan and a full panel of blood tests—appropriately, I thought. He was probably checking for something else that could account for her symptoms—evidence of a small stroke, a brain tumor, or thyroid abnormalities. But then he did something I could not fathom: He called Sister Laura and told her—over the phone—that she appeared to have the early signs of Alzheimer's disease.

"I was devastated," she recalled. After doing her best to pull herself together, she decided to talk with her biological sister, who was a few years younger and also a School Sister of Notre Dame. Her sister assured Sister Laura that, no matter what, she would always love and care for her. "That was a huge relief," said Sister Laura. But she ignored her sister's recommendation that she seek a second opinion, accepting her doctor's judgment that her mind was beginning to fail. "That's life," she concluded.

Sister Laura felt obliged to inform the other sisters in her small convent about her newly diagnosed condition. "Some of them started to check on me for the most routine things," she recalled, shaking her head. "When I would use the stove, they would come in afterward to see whether I had shut off the burners.

"Dr. Snowdon, do you know what my worst fear was?" Now her eyes started to well up with tears. "That I was going to forget Jesus," she said. "I finally realized that I may not remember Him, but He will remember me."

One sister who knew Sister Laura well insisted that there was nothing wrong with her mind. But even though her depression had lifted somewhat, Sister Laura had become hyperaware of every occasion on which her memory failed her, every lapse in her attention. She remained convinced that she had Alzheimer's and that it was slowly progressing. Four years after her diagnosis, a nurse overheard her telling another sister about her condition. "Excuse me, Sister Laura, that's not possible," the nurse said.

Sister Laura carefully explained to the nurse that she had not dreamed this up: A doctor had made the diagnosis. With the nurse's encouragement, Sister Laura finally sought a second opinion and underwent a thorough medical and psychological evaluation. (Most cities in the United States now have specialized medical teams—as at the University of Kentucky Memory Disorders Clinic—that work together to diagnose Alzheimer's.) Sister Laura was examined by a neurologist, who assessed her physical signs and symptoms, checked her blood chemistry, and did another brain scan. She also took a comprehensive battery of psychological tests. At the end of this workup, she was relieved to learn that her mind was completely intact.

Because of a doctor's misdiagnosis, Sister Laura had suffered unnecessarily for four years. While I do not think that my mistake with Sister Louise was as egregious, the parallels disturbed me and forced me to think long and hard about this brave new genetic world we have entered.

━

In 1997 I visited the Duke University lab of neurologist Allen Roses, the controversial researcher who with his colleagues had discovered the link between APOE-4 and Alzheimer's—in my opinion, the most important Alzheimer's breakthrough in the last half of the twentieth century. Roses had a humorous perspective on his own reputation. Shortly before my visit, he had testified at a Senate subcommittee hearing on aging. "I have been personally called a number of things," he told the senators. "Maverick" and "street fighter" were two of the "more favorable," he noted.

I got along fine with Roses, and I enjoyed his flair. A couple of years earlier, Roses had generously done APOE-4 genotyping on 619 sisters in the Nun Study. Consistent with other studies of Caucasian populations, we found that 20 percent (125) of the sisters had one copy of the APOE-4 gene, while only 2.6 percent (16) had two APOE-4 genes. (The percentages for African Americans and other ethnic groups are still being debated.)

Now we were planning additional ways to utilize the Nun Study genetic data in our research. After we had agreed on our next steps, Roses said that he had a proposition for me: He would write me a check for $200 if I could find a cognitively intact sister with two copies of the APOE-4 gene who had reached her ninetieth birthday.

Roses' challenge amused me. I knew it was a standing offer he'd made to other researchers—his way of insisting on the power of the APOE-4 gene. Nobody had collected on his bet to date, but maybe I was the one. While findings from the Nun Study—and numerous other studies around the world—had shown that these genes greatly increased the risk of Alzheimer's, I also knew that even two APOE-4 genes had not produced Alzheimer's symptoms in all of our study participants. So I booted up my laptop, extremely proud of the cognitive abilities of many of the oldest sisters in the Nun Study—and hoping to find the exception to his rule.

I homed in on the sixteen double-APOE-4 sisters and found that four had lived past their ninetieth birthday. Three of these women had shown cognitive impairments by one of our main measures, the Mini-Mental State Exam: They had scored under 24 out of a possible 30 points, the cutoff point for normal. But the fourth sister had a 26. "I've got one!" I announced.

Roses looked surprised. "How much education did she have?" he quickly asked.

I sifted through the database again and found that she had earned a master's degree.

"Well, given her high level of education, here at Duke we would require someone like her to have more than twenty-six points on the MMSE to qualify as cognitively intact."

So according to Roses' system of handicapping, I had lost. However, I had to agree with him about holding this highly educated sister to a higher standard on the MMSE, because our own findings suggested the protective effects of education. But as much respect as I have for Roses, I remained skeptical about his assertion that two APOE-4 genes *always* cause the disease by age ninety. To be precise, I didn't want to believe it. Genes behave differently in different people, and already we have seen great variances in our double-APOE-4 sisters. I am convinced that the Nun Study still has much to teach us on this score.

Back in 1986 I put in some long days and weeks when I began studying the Mankato sisters, but nothing like the schedule Rudolph Tanzi was keeping. The young scientist at Harvard Medical School was regularly spending twelve to fifteen hours a day in the lab trying to break the genetic code for Alzheimer's disease. As Tanzi later recalled in an interview in the *New York Times,* when he felt he was close to the solution, he worked all night on Christmas Eve, the entire day of Christmas, all of New Year's Eve, and again through the next day. "It was obsession," he acknowledged, ruefully noting that it had ruined his marriage. But it also made scientific history.

The following year, two back-to-back articles appeared in the prestigious journal *Science.* The lead author of one of those articles was Tanzi; the lead author of the other was Dmitry Goldgaber, then of the National Institutes of Health. Both articles identified the same gene for Alzheimer's disease. Unlike Roses' 1992 discovery of the APOE-4 gene's relationship to late-onset Alzheimer's, Tanzi and Goldgaber had isolated a gene involved in the much rarer early-onset form of the disease.

Early-onset Alzheimer's typically strikes before the age of sixty-five and spreads through families much more predictably than the late-onset variety. It accounts for something like 5 to 10 percent of all Alzheimer's cases. It also afflicts people with Down syndrome; nearly everyone with that condition develops extensive plaques and tangles by the age of fifty. Since people with Down syndrome have an extra copy of chromosome 21, the researchers reasoned that they would be more susceptible to any gene it carried. This had led them to focus their search on chromosome 21.

As the articles in *Science* reported, the gene for amyloid (the stuff of plaques) had been found on chromosome 21. As it turned out, the gene coded for a much larger protein—dubbed the beta-amyloid precursor protein, or APP—and people with Alzheimer's disease and Down syndrome did not, as first imagined, simply make more of it. Rather, the trouble arose when the amyloid was cut out of the larger precursor protein by enzymes in the body.

In the presence of normal amyloid, neurons function just fine. If the APP is improperly cut, however, the resulting amyloid becomes sticky and clumps together, forming plaques. These plaques are toxic to neurons. They also appear to stimulate the immune system to mount an inflammatory response, which further damages the neurons. In turn, the theory holds, this mayhem causes a chemical reaction that leads to the tangles inside the nerve cells. The entire toxic domino effect has been dubbed the amyloid cascade hypothesis.

There later turned out to be three genes that, in mutant form, contribute to plaque formation: not only the APP gene, but also presenilin 1, on chromosome 14, and presenilin 2, on chromosome 1. Unlike the APOE-4 gene, these genes occur rarely—less than 1 percent of the population has any one of them.

As Tanzi recounts in *Decoding Darkness,* his book about his research, the amyloid cascade hypothesis has been bolstered by several mouse studies. Mice engineered to carry a mutated APP gene went on to develop an extraordinarily high number of plaques in their brains. In 1999 the genetically engineered mice were given a vaccine containing the noxious form of amyloid. In young mice, this triggered production of antibodies that appeared to prevent the development of plaques. In older mice, which had already developed plaques, vaccination markedly slowed the formation of new plaques. There was excited speculation that an amyloid-based vaccine might be able to treat as well as prevent Alzheimer's.

Tanzi and many other scientists have come to view amyloid, or plaques, as the main culprit in Alzheimer's disease. But Allen Roses looked at the disease from an entirely different perspective—possibly due, in part, to his focus on the far more common form of late-onset Alzheimer's. Together with a handful of other prominent researchers, he challenged the amyloid cascade hypothesis with an alternative possibility: that the tau protein that makes up the tangles better explains how Alzheimer's damages the brain.

The tau hypothesis rests in part on the famous autopsy studies of Braak and Braak, which showed that tangles and their location could be used to map the stages of the disease. It also rests on the argument, outlined in Chapter 6, about how the tangles are formed. Tau makes up the ropelike microtubules in normal neurons, but there are abnormal forms of tau that can tangle the ropes. Roses contended that APOE-3, the most common form of the gene, prevents these tangles from forming, while APOE-4 provides no protection against tangling. Roses also believes that APOE-4 helps spur plaque formation.

Sorting out the relationship of Alzheimer's disease to amyloid and tau, plaques and tangles, is a confusing task that over the years has caused major rifts between the competing groups of researchers. In the Alzheimer's field, the two sides are jokingly called the Tauists and the Baptists (from beta-amyloid protein), like participants in some holy war.

The central dilemma, as is often the case in scientific studies (and in epidemiology in particular), is separating cause from effect. Do toxic pieces of beta-amyloid, as the Baptists believe, trigger a cascade of events that obliterate neurons? Or is the buildup of amyloid plaques simply an effect—what the Tauists call a tombstone, a marker of the nerve cell death caused by dangerous forms of tau?

This is far from an ivory-tower debate between the high priests of the Baptist and Tauist faithful. Understanding the precise mechanisms by which plaques and tangles are formed might lead to vaccines and drugs that can prevent and treat this terrible disease. (Both Roses and Tanzi are involved in the search for practical applications of their research—Roses at the pharmaceutical giant GlaxoSmithKline, and Tanzi through his interest in a company called Prana Biotechnology.) Following the wrong road can cost years of research time and result in a lost opportunity to prevent enormous suffering.

My own thinking leans toward the Tauists, partly as a result of what I have learned at consensus conferences on more than 250 brains. Our Nun Study data show a strong correlation between the number and distribution of tangles in Markesbery's pathology reports and the results of our mental and physical evaluations—a far stronger correlation than they do for the number of plaques. But I retain an open mind about the cause—or, more likely, the *causes*—of Alzheimer's. As researchers clarify the relationship between Alzheimer's genes and what we see in the brain under the microscope, I am confident that the pieces of the puzzle will fall into place. Until then, it's important to keep in mind that our genes are hardly the only factor determining our fate.

—

The sisters I will call Joyce, Bernadette, and Suzanne each inherited two copies of the APOE-4 gene. The three School Sisters of Notre Dame were nearly the same age, all having been born in the early 1910s. Each came from a large, working-class family, and none of their parents had more than an eighth-grade education. Each had earned a master's degree and worked as a teacher for more than forty years. Yet that is where the similarities ended.

Sister Joyce represents a textbook clinical case of a double APOE-4 gene. We first tested Sister Joyce in 1992, when she was in her late seventies. She scored a perfect 30 on the Mini-Mental State Exam and needed no assistance with any of the activities of daily living, like walking, dressing, or feeding herself. In Sister Joyce's Delayed Word Recall test, which gauges short-term memory, she remembered five of the ten words she had learned five minutes earlier.

By Sister Joyce's second annual evaluation, we could see clear hints of a decline in some of her tests. Notable was a drop in the Delayed Word Recall, where she was able to remember only three of the ten words. By her third evaluation, she had declined in virtually every mental and physical test we administered.

Still, she did not meet our criteria for dementia, and a linguistic sample—a test in which we ask sisters to write for ten minutes about their lives before they entered the convent—documents that Sister Joyce could still communicate effectively:

I had a wish to be a nun because of Sister Mary John, my
aunt. Mother did not wish me to join the SSND because

they were strict and did not allow sisters to go home for va-cations. My Dad was glad to have me join the SSND's, since that is where his sister, Sr. Mary John, was.

People with dementia typically cannot write so lucidly.

Sister Joyce's next evaluation took place when she was in her mid-eighties. By now she had crossed the line: Her MMSE score had plummeted to 11 out of a possible 30 points, and she could not remember any of the ten words on the Delayed Word Recall test. By this time she also needed assistance in simple tasks such as dressing and getting out of a chair. Her linguistic sample was particularly telling. Here is what she wrote, in its entirety:

Short description of life before I entered convent. My place of birth, parantage school attended. What, caused good family meals and father's love. What influenzed me to be-come a sister when my father encouraged me.

Sister Gabriel Mary, who administered this test, included the following comment in her research notes: "Sister wrote well beyond the 10 minutes and clearly wanted to finish the last sentence. She was as far as the word 'father' and took 4 or 5 minutes trying to think of the next word she wanted."

At Sister Joyce's next exam, she left the linguistic sample completely blank. "Sister held the pen in her right hand for al-most 2 minutes," noted Sister Gabriel Mary. "I thought she might attempt to write, but after some time she put the pen down and shoved the paper away from her."

Sister Gabriel Mary did note, however, that Sister Joyce looked at her when she spoke, smiled, and even laughed once. As of this writing, Sister Joyce requires full-time nursing assis-tance and still manages to smile from time to time.

Now consider the history of Sister Bernadette. When she was in her early eighties, sixty years after she joined the congregation, Sister Bernadette took her first Nun Study examination. She scored high in every category, including a perfect 30 on the MMSE, and needed absolutely no help performing the activities of daily living. During her next two exams, there was no evidence of decline in any of the mental or physical tests. In 1996, when Sister Bernadette was eighty-five, she passed away from a heart attack—and we were in for some surprises.

As I noted in Chapter 6, an autopsy of Sister Bernadette's brain revealed that tangles had riddled her hippocampus and neocortex, so much so that Markesbery ranked her as a Braak stage VI. This indicated severe Alzheimer's pathology and was completely consistent with her double APOE-4 status. Yet Sister Bernadette had shown no symptoms of dementia whatsoever. In fact, when we held the consensus conference following her autopsy, we were so dumbfounded by her lack of symptoms that we feared UPS had shipped us the wrong brain.

However, her double APOE-4 status cross-checked with the data from Roses' lab. And any doubt about her reported mental status was eliminated when we watched her incredible performance on the videotapes of her last three exams before her death. At each exam she had performed the feat of estimating the time of day within four minutes of the clock on our computer.

To date, Sister Bernadette has the distinction of being the only Braak stage VI in the entire Nun Study who remained entirely intact, both mentally and physically, on all our tests. Despite her severe brain pathology and double APOE-4 status, she had apparently evaded the symptoms of Alzheimer's by dying before her brain was overwhelmed. Had she lived longer, I suspect that Alzheimer's would have started to chip away at her memories and other abilities—but we will never know. Sister Bernadette stands as a testament to what is possible in resisting the genetic and pathological forces of Alzheimer's.

Only one other sister in our study who had two copies of the APOE-4 gene died—or "escaped," as the researchers say—before she developed the symptoms of Alzheimer's disease. Nine sisters with a double dose of APOE-4 developed dementia, and four others had short-term memory problems before they died. This leaves only one of the sixteen sisters in our study with a double APOE-4 gene unaccounted for. And, like Sister Bernadette, she is remarkable.

We have evaluated Sister Suzanne six times, beginning when she was in her late seventies. Her most recent exam, when she was in her mid-eighties, showed no evidence of any cognitive or physical impairments—not even a hint of a problem.

I of course have no idea whether Sister Suzanne's brain has been invaded by plaques and tangles, or whether she will develop symptoms later on. But given what I have seen of her performance to date, I suspect that she may make it to age ninety perfectly intact. I would be delighted for her, and I would be happy to report this to Allen Roses and see him take out his checkbook to pay off his bet.

—

In 1995, after Allen Roses had offered to screen the Nun Study sisters for the APOE-4 gene, I visited each convent to explain this new phase of our research to the participants. On one afternoon I met with about thirty sisters in a former chapel at Elm Grove that had been converted into a library. In the soft light coming in through the stained-glass windows, I described to the sisters how we would, with their permission, take a sample for genotyping. We would simply swab the inside of their cheeks with a small brush, and this would pick up a few old cells that were naturally shed from the lining of the mouth. This would allow us to test for the APOE-4 gene, and we would also freeze the remaining genetic material for future analysis. As new "candidate" genes were discovered, we would defrost minute samples of their genetic material and reexamine it to see how the newly identified genes related to the pathology and symptoms of Alzheimer's. In conclusion, I assured the sisters that the results would be completely confidential.

In the question period that followed, several sisters voiced their concern that someone else would know their genetic status—and their potential risk of developing the disease. One sister asked, "Will you tell us if we have the gene?" I replied that they could have the information if they requested it—but I also wanted to deflect the issue. "If your faculties are so keen that you can even think about such concerns, then you probably have nothing to worry about," I said. I knew this was glib as soon as it was out of my mouth. But the sisters, polite as always, let the matter drop.

Four years later I again sat in that library at Elm Grove with many of the same sisters. Joining me this time was Dr. Piero Antuono from the Medical College of Wisconsin, who was about to conduct neurological evaluations of the sisters that we would add to our data. We had nearly finished discussing our recent findings when Sister Rosalie asked, "I sometimes have difficulty remembering the names of sisters I've known for years. Do you think I am getting Alzheimer's disease?"

"Well, Sister, I'm only in my forties," I answered, "and I sometimes blank out on the name of a friend, or walk into a room and can't remember why I'm there, or can't immediately come up with the name of an object. This kind of thing can happen at any age. A lot of it is due to stress or anxiety or fatigue or trying to pay attention to too many things at the same time. It's also normal that as we get older, we need a bit more time to process things. Many people can't remember a name on the spot, but it comes to them later.

"What is not normal is when these memory problems persist and progressively get worse. That's the time to seek medical attention. But remember, even then, the difficulty could be due to a side effect from a medication you are taking, or something else that could be treated. We've had people consult us about a relative who kept asking the same questions, and the real problem turned out to be hearing loss." I could see Sister Rosalie, and several other sisters around her, let out a collective sigh of relief.

Then Sister Berenice spoke up. "I'd like to know what you found out about my genes—whether or not I have the Alzheimer's gene." Both Piero and I shifted uncomfortably in our chairs. Piero was the first to respond.

"Before I address that directly, Sister, I'd like to make an important point. Genes certainly play a role in who gets Alzheimer's—although I don't believe we've found all the genes involved. But the more we learn about genes in general, the more we realize that most of them interact with lifestyle and environment. You've heard about the nature-versus-nurture debate. We're now finding that it's more like nature *plus* nurture.

"Genes seem to be very important in early-onset Alzheimer's. But for late-onset Alzheimer's—the only kind you need to worry about—we're finding other factors. I like to emphasize things people can do something about, such as avoiding smoking and head trauma—always wear your seat belt!—or taking certain vitamins and antioxidants, or maintaining their cardiovascular health. There are good reasons for doing these things anyway—and in addition, they may help to prevent Alzheimer's.

"Now, to get back to your original question. I'd like to ask you one thing: Would knowing that you had a gene for Alzheimer's really change what you did day-to-day? Would it really help you make better decisions?"

I chimed in. "It's not as though you'd need to get your life in order if you discovered you had the gene. It gives you a certain probability of something happening down the line, but it tells you very little about your immediate future." To me, of course, the sisters already seemed to have their lives completely in order, but even for the rest of us, there are far more urgent reasons to make a will or reconcile past hurts with family and friends.

It was Piero's question—in essence, "What difference would it make if you knew?"—that seemed to resonate the most with the sisters. I repeated it when the issue came up at the other convents, and it seemed to resolve their anxieties in a very direct and practical way.

Someday very soon, however, I will probably have to change my tune. Tanzi, Roses, and many other respected scientists believe that within five to ten years there will be drugs that can slow the development of Alzheimer's lesions and prevent their damage to the brain. And probably six to a dozen other genes in addition to APOE-4 will be confirmed as true risk factors for late-onset Alzheimer's, which makes up about 90 percent of all Alzheimer's cases worldwide. Sometime during this decade we will probably be able to test for this battery of genes and develop more reliable predictions of who truly is at risk for late-onset disease. Then, given the promise of combining pharmacology with genetics, we will ultimately be able to tailor individual combinations of drugs to target specific genetic and biological imbalances.

When that day comes, we are in for an immense national debate—as is already going on in other areas. Suppose millions of middle-aged people discover that their genome puts them at risk for Alzheimer's and that they can avoid the disease by taking several drugs daily for the rest of their lives. The social, legal, economic, and ethical issues this raises are simply staggering.

The potential for genetic discrimination is also huge. How will friends and family, bosses and coworkers, and doctors and nurses—not to mention the accountants at our HMOs—respond to the news that we are genetically at risk for Alzheimer's? This concern was brought home to me right after the *Journal of the American Medical Association* published our paper on the autobiographies. Within a few days—to my utter astonishment—we were deluged by calls from insurance companies that wanted us to develop a standardized pen-and-paper test for susceptibility to Alzheimer's. We firmly declined—but the point had been indelibly made.

Over the coming years, as we, in Tanzi's words, continue to "decode darkness," our challenge will be to keep in mind that genetic information is a double-edged sword, equally capable of illuminating the way and, if used improperly, darkening our lives.

9

———— ✦ ————

The Heart of the Matter

When I knock on a door, I never know what a sister will be
doing or how she is feeling. So while I am walking to her room,
I pray to the Holy Spirit to guide me as to what to say, what
questions I should ask, or whether I should just
listen for a while.

—Sister Marlene Manney

At the Mankato convent in November 1992 we gave Sister Agnes what would be the first and last mental exam she would take as part of the Nun Study.

"Sister, can you hear me?" asked Sister Gabriel Mary Spaeth, the examiner.

Sister Agnes, who was ninety-two, kept her eyes closed, as she would for most of the exam, occasionally opening them when she heard her name.

Sister Gabriel Mary was using our special protocol to assess Sister Agnes. She had already determined, in her gentle way, that Sister Agnes could not respond to the demands of our regular assessment of mental and physical abilities. The special protocol gives us a way to assess the most basic mental function: the ability to respond to communication and stimuli. Because the special protocol looks for the smallest flickers of response in the person being tested, it requires great patience from the examiner and what often seem like repetitive questions. The test is standardized by design, but Sister Gabriel Mary infuses it with a very personal sense of compassion and reassurance.

"Sister, squeeze my hand," said Sister Gabriel Mary. Sister Agnes, a frail woman who was a few inches shy of five feet tall and barely weighed a hundred pounds, sat passively. At long last this former organist and music teacher gave a squeeze with her right hand. But when Sister Gabriel Mary asked her to use her left hand, she did not move it from where it lay on the table.

Sister Gabriel Mary then showed Sister Agnes a bright yellow ball. "Sister?" she asked. "What is this?" And then she waited, giving her a chance to process the question.

Sister Agnes looked at the yellow ball in Sister Gabriel Mary's hand. She reached for it but did not say anything.

After some time Sister Gabriel Mary repeated, "What is this?" Noting that Sister Agnes' eyes were closed, she gently touched her arm and added, "Look at this, Sister."

After thirty more seconds of silence, Sister Gabriel Mary said, "This is a ball. What is this?"

Another long silence.

—

Sister Agnes was a "century baby," born in 1900. She grew up on a midwestern farm, the last of eleven children, and abandoned her studies after the eighth grade to care for her invalid father and help her mother run the house. In her spare time she gave a hand at the local Catholic church, washing the altar linens, decorating the altar, and ringing the Angelus bell to call parishioners to prayer. "I enjoyed doing all this work for the Lord," she later wrote in her autobiography. Her father died when she was eighteen, but she stayed on to help her mother until, at the relatively advanced age of twenty-three, she decided to join the School Sisters of Notre Dame.

After professing her vows, Sister Agnes played the organ and taught music at churches and schools around Minnesota and North Dakota, spending summers at the Mankato provincial house in order to attend high school classes. She was awarded her diploma at age twenty-eight. After more than fifty years of service, she returned to Good Counsel Hill to retire. Several years later she moved into the St. Joseph's health-care wing of the convent, where nurses cared for sisters who had pronounced physical or mental problems. As I had discovered during my earliest visits to Mankato, this nursing-home-within-a-convent allowed the sisters not only to receive excellent medical care, but to remain in familiar surroundings and enjoy the support and spirit of their community.

Sister Agnes' medical records detailed the convergence of three problems: stroke, heart disease, and dementia. How these three diseases overlap—and how they are linked to Alzheimer's—became a key focus of the Nun Study. We knew from the outset that stroke and heart disease significantly increase a person's risk of developing dementia. What was less clear was the *kind* of dementia involved and how it is triggered in the brain.

Strokes can bring on the sudden appearance of dementia symptoms that are caused by the rupture or blockage of a blood vessel. In contrast, the symptoms of Alzheimer's disease usually progress slowly. However, with advancing age, these two diseases may become intertwined and confused. How stroke and Alzheimer's knot together is far from an academic question. Effective prevention and treatment strategies might result from untying that knot.

—

Sister Gabriel Mary Spaeth and Sister Marlene Manney joined the Nun Study in 1991, just as our testing program was getting under way. For eleven months of the year they are on the road in their Plymouth Grand Voyager minivan, visiting each Nun Study participant in each of the seven Notre Dame provinces in the United States. During their visits Sisters Gabriel Mary and Marlene carefully evaluate the mental and physical abilities of the sisters, using special tests that they have helped us refine. Because these two sisters look so much alike—they are both about five foot four, with similar hairstyles and glasses, and even similar smiles—they have become affectionately known as the Snowdon Sisters or the Snowdon Twins. (They wear name tags during their visits so that the other sisters can more easily tell them apart.) The Nun Study could not exist without them. They supply us with our lifeblood: information about how our participants change over time.

The sisters' year usually starts in Milwaukee, Sister Gabriel Mary's home province. After doing assessments in that region for three months, they move on to Sister Marlene's home province, Mankato, for about two months. Then they journey to Chicago, St. Louis, Chatawa, Baltimore, Wilton, and back to Milwaukee.

Their minivan is jam-packed with assessment tools, including computers, printers, tape recorders and video cameras, a walker, and boxes of files. Gifts made by study participants have also become part of the regular cargo: a wreath from St. Louis that hangs by the rearview mirror, a dashboard cloth doll from Baltimore, and two stuffed animals (a rabbit and a bear) from the Chatawa convent.

Their days on the road begin in prayer. The sister who is not driving reads aloud the prayer and the Mass reading for the day. Then they remain quiet for the first hour or so, reflecting on the day's scripture and how it applies to their lives. "This sets the tone for my day," Sister Gabriel Mary once told me. "Then as occasions arise during the day, I turn to God with a silent prayer."

Later in the morning they sometimes play music, and one of them often crochets while the other drives. (One of the bonuses of their travel, Sister Marlene says, is collecting new crochet patterns from sisters at different convents.) Usually night has fallen before they reach the next convent—or, if necessary, check into a Holiday Inn.

Each arrival at a convent is something of a homecoming, as they greet their friends, catch up on local events and find out what birthdays and jubilees (vows anniversaries) are to be celebrated during their time there. After they unpack their van—their least-favorite activity—Sisters Marlene and Gabriel Mary meet with all the Nun Study participants to update them about our most recent research findings. They then review the assessment process with the sisters, stressing that the evaluations are for research only. "It's a natural aging process if you cannot walk as quickly as you did the last time we visited," Sister Marlene reassures the sisters. "If there were no changes," Sister Gabriel Mary adds, "then there would be no point to doing the research."

For each participant, the mental assessment is done one day, followed by the physical assessment the next. The sisters conduct five or six evaluations each day, audiotaping all of them and videotaping many. Preparation and follow-up work fill the remainder of the busy day.

The mental evaluation includes eight different but overlapping tests. Many of them would be familiar to anyone who has witnessed a diagnostic workup for suspected Alzheimer's. The Mini-Mental State Examination asks the sister being tested to name specific objects, state the date, identify her location, spell words backward, and do other simple tasks. This helps us assess important components of overall mental function such as memory, concentration, and orientation to time and place.

The participant's ability to recognize and name common objects is assessed by two other tests. (Recall that one of the symptoms Alois Alzheimer noted was that his patient, Auguste D., called a cup a "milk pourer.") The test called Boston Naming asks the sister to name fifteen objects depicted in line drawings on large index cards. Since some sisters might fail this test because of poor visual acuity, another test, called Object Naming, allows them to use their hands to identify a different set of twelve real items.

The next test, called Verbal Fluency, measures language, memory, and processing speed. Participants are asked to name as many items in a given class, such as fruits and vegetables, as they can in one minute. Another test, called Constructional Praxis, measures visual-spatial ability: Sisters are shown four line drawings of geometrical shapes and asked to copy them.

All of these tests are designed to locate the participant somewhere on a spectrum of ability. For example, the Constructional Praxis test asks sisters to draw shapes of increasing complexity. The objects depicted in Boston Naming range from the common to the less frequently encountered. All the abilities being tested relate to those needed for everyday tasks and are important for maintaining independence.

The final three memory tests build on each other. First there is Word List Memory, in which the participant reads aloud ten words three times and then immediately is asked to recall them. This is the learning phase of the test, and it is repeated three times, with the ten words arranged differently each time. Five minutes later, in the Delayed Word Recall test, the participant is asked to recollect the ten words. Finally, in the Word Recognition test, twenty large index cards are shown to the participant. Ten of the cards contain the learned words and the other ten contain "distracter" words—words the participant has not previously encountered during the testing. The task is to distinguish the learned words from the distracter words.

About 75 percent of the sisters are able to correctly recognize more of the learned words on the Word Recognition test than they could remember in the Word Recall test. This difference demonstrates the importance of the visual component of memory, and explains why visual cues—such as the name tags Sisters Gabriel Mary and Marlene wear—can help those with faltering memories.

The physical tests attempt to mimic real-world tasks. Sisters are asked to put on a sweater, cut a clay hot dog, and read the instructions on a pill bottle and take out the correct dosage. Hand coordination is tested by timing the sisters as they open three small doors with different latches, and grip strength is measured by a device called a dynamometer that the sisters squeeze. The evaluator times how long it takes each participant to walk six feet and, if they are able, fifty feet. The participants are also timed on the Up-and-Go test, where they are asked to stand up and walk around a stop sign that is kept at each convent for the tests. Lower-body strength is indirectly measured by determining how high the sister can step onto a platform. For this test we use the kind of adjustable-height platform designed for step aerobics classes. The participant is also asked to put on a pair of shoes and tie them. (Before the study began, we purchased twelve pairs of the same style of shoes in different sizes so that we could standardize this test.)

All of these performance-based tests are supplemented by reports from the convent's nursing staff on the participants' ability during the preceding six months to accomplish the activities of daily living, such as eating, dressing, getting to the toilet, and bathing. It is when a sister clearly cannot perform these mental and physical tests that the evaluator uses our special protocol—as Sister Gabriel Mary did with Sister Agnes.

During all of our assessments, the evaluators accentuate the positive, complimenting the participants for their accomplishments, whether it is acing the Delayed Word Recall test or simply squeezing a hand during the special-protocol testing. This is especially crucial for the more disabled sisters, who understandably are particularly sensitive to the emotional tone of the evaluation. The participants often report to me that they appreciate how quickly Sisters Gabriel Mary and Marlene put them at ease—a testament to both our evaluators' technical skills and to their good hearts.

—

When I received the special-protocol results for Sister Agnes, I reviewed her records and discovered that she was one of the sixteen classmates who in 1927 took first vows with Sister Nicolette—"the last nun standing." Unfortunately, age had not been as kind to Sister Agnes. She appears with Sister Nicolette in the sixtieth-anniversary photo, taken in 1987, when ten members of the vows class were still alive, but her physical and mental function had already declined sharply by that time.

Sister Agnes had a history of strokes and ministrokes that dated back to 1955. In 1977 she had undefined heart trouble, and in 1983 a doctor noted that she probably had suffered an undetected heart attack. By this time her circulatory problems were affecting both the nerve tissue in her brain and the muscles in her heart.

Sister Agnes fell several times in her eighties, sometimes after becoming dizzy or light-headed, and she began to use a walker regularly. These attacks of dizziness may have been symptoms of ministrokes, called transient ischemic attacks (TIAs). TIAs, which sometimes last only a few minutes (and not more than twenty-four hours), signal that parts of the brain have become temporarily ischemic—that is, they are not receiving enough blood flow or oxygen. TIAs may be an early warning sign of impending stroke, which causes permanent damage to the brain, with symptoms lasting more than twenty-four hours.

Stroke and heart disease often have similar, overlapping causes. High blood pressure is the most important factor. When a person has high blood pressure, or hypertension, the heart must work overtime to pump blood, which also increases the risk of congestive heart failure and heart attack. In the brain, hypertension can lead to the blockage and rupture of an artery, producing a stroke—which essentially is a brain attack.

The other main threat to the heart and the brain is atherosclerosis, the process by which fatty deposits form plaques on the interior walls of the blood vessels. These clogged vessels cannot carry as much blood and thus reduce the supply of oxygen and nutrients to the body's tissues and organs. The heart responds by pumping more blood, sometimes stressing this vital muscle to the point that it becomes inefficient—even though it's working overtime.

Nothing loves oxygen more than the brain, which accounts for only about 2 percent of the body's weight but demands 15 to 25 percent of the available oxygen. The hippocampus, which is so critical to memory, is particularly sensitive to ischemic damage. So the brain literally chokes when a compromised heart or a clogged artery cannot deliver enough oxygen-loaded blood. Hypertension again comes into play here, as extra pressure on the walls of arteries stiffens them, making it easier for fatty plaques to form.

Whichever culprit starves the brain of oxygen, the result is often the same: stroke. First nerve cells die. Then, in a second wave of insult and injury, the brain tissue becomes inflamed. This initiates the so-called inflammatory cascade, in which the cells release toxic chemicals, killing more brain cells and further damaging the blood vessels. Depending on the location of the damage, the results may include partial paralysis, impaired vision, loss of speech—and what is called vascular dementia.

—

What is this?" Sister Gabriel Mary asked slowly, holding up a doll for Sister Agnes to see. After repeating the question without any response, she said, "Sister, this is a doll. What is this?"

Again Sister Agnes did not respond.

Sister Gabriel Mary then took a harmonica from her box of test equipment and blew a few notes. "Do you hear that, Sister?" she asked playfully.

Sister Agnes nodded—yes.

Encouraged, Sister Gabriel Mary held out the harmonica to her. "What is that?" she asked, hoping that Sister Agnes would reach for it.

But Sister Agnes remained silent, and her hands did not move.

—

One month after Sister Agnes turned eighty-seven, nurses began to make detailed notes about the ups and downs of her mental status. Any dementing disease is a roller-coaster ride of hope and despair, both for those suffering its symptoms and for those who provide care. I felt heartsick just reading Sister Agnes' medical charts.

"Needs supervision so she doesn't wander off, as she becomes confused at times," wrote a nurse in February 1987. The next month a nurse noted that Sister Agnes no longer had complaints of dizziness and "appears to be more organized regarding time and place, periods of confusion less." A month later she was "taking advantage of the nice weather" and going outside for walks by herself. That May, however, a nurse noted that Sister Agnes "needs to be watched more closely as she tries walking stairs with walker." In June she fell in the hallway and required a total hip replacement. Her mental condition began to deteriorate rapidly.

By 1988 Sister Agnes needed help with basic self-care. A nurse noted in March that Sister Agnes remained "pleasant, quiet, alert" but also that she had a "memory span of short periods" and had slipped to the floor and lacerated her head. "Forgetful at times," wrote a nurse two months later. In July a nurse noted that "some days she is more confused than others."

At the start of 1989 Sister Agnes was still reading the newspaper each day, visiting the convent grounds with her walker, and slowly strolling to the dining room and the chapel. But that April Sister Agnes had what a nurse described as "a slight stroke" and began to lean to her left side. She soon began using a wheelchair as well as a walker, and the weakness on her left side became more pronounced.

—

Sister, make a fist," said Sister Gabriel Mary.

Sister Agnes made a fist with her right hand.

"Good!" said Sister Gabriel Mary, who sounded surprised and elated at the response.

But Sister Agnes could not make a fist with her left hand.

Sister Gabriel Mary then touched Sister Agnes' right leg. "Sister, move this leg," she said. Sister Agnes sat still. She did not react when Sister Gabriel Mary touched her left leg, either.

—

By 1990 Sister Agnes had become confused "a lot of the time," wrote one nurse. She had bad bouts with diarrhea, and the nurses often would find her in the bathroom, her chart noted in July. By October Sister Agnes had become more dependent on her wheelchair.

In June 1991 a nurse noted, "Not oriented to time and date. Does not engage in much conversation." By November Sister Agnes could not swallow pureed food. However, in January 1992, the month she turned ninety-two, she had her last teeth removed, and a nurse commented, "Sister has become more like her old self, smiling, chatting, eating pureed food." Still, the overall course was downward.

—

Sister, look," said Gabriel Mary, showing her the yellow ball that she had used at the beginning of the assessment. "Do you see it?"

Sister Gabriel Mary got up and walked across the room, waving the ball as she went. Sister Agnes' eyes followed her, confirming that she could see at a distance. It was not her vision that had failed her.

Returning to Sister Agnes' side, Sister Gabriel Mary took her hand. "Sister Agnes, thank you for coming in today to help us. What you have done will help many people. I will keep you in my prayers."

During the special protocol, Sister Gabriel Mary had filled out a form that assessed Sister Agnes' ability to perform each task, circling either *yes* or *no* next to each one attempted. Sister Gabriel Mary circled *no* thirty out of thirty-five times.

I once asked Sister Gabriel Mary how such a trying assessment makes her feel. "Often after working with a special-protocol participant, I reflect in awe at the working of the human brain, its puzzlement, and I wonder, what was really going on in this sister's mind?" Sister Gabriel Mary told me. "How much of what I said did she comprehend? How frustrating it must be for her to understand me but not to be able to communicate her thoughts to me in a way I could understand. I feel strongly that regardless of how confused a sister may appear, she has times of cognizant recognition or realization of what is going on." Empathy like this has to be one of the reasons that the Snowdon Sisters have been able to avoid burnout.

———

In late November, ten days after Sister Gabriel Mary's special-protocol evaluation, a nurse observed that Sister Agnes was sleeping much of the time and "even needs to be coaxed to open her eyes." Come Christmas Eve, Sister Agnes developed a cold and became extremely congested, with loud rales emanating from her lungs each time she took a breath. Just before the year ended, a nurse filled in the bottom of the last page in Sister Agnes' chart. "Sister appeared comatose this evening," she wrote. "Sister died peacefully 6 P.M. RIP." At 6 P.M., Mankato's Angelus bell rang for evening prayers.

On Sister Agnes' death certificate, the cause of death was stated as "CVA," shorthand for cerebrovascular accident, better known as a stroke. But what was the cause of her dementia? As a Nun Study participant, Sister Agnes had agreed to donate her brain upon death, and this gave us the opportunity to perform a detailed investigation into a question that too often goes unanswered.

Sister Agnes' brain arrived at Bill Markesbery's lab at the Center on Aging shortly after she died. Markesbery did not need his microscope to see the damage done by her strokes. Their impact on the white matter of her brain was evident even on the gross exam, the physical inspection made with the naked eye.

The white matter lies just beneath the gray matter of the brain and is partly composed of the long "tail," or axon, that extends out from the soma, or main cell body, of each neuron. The gray soma contains the neuron's genetic matter and its central processing functions; the axon—which can range from a fraction of an inch to a couple of feet in length—relays the neuron's messages to other neurons throughout the brain and body. A white fatty substance called myelin acts as a protective sheath around the axon, much like the plastic coating on an electrical wire. The white matter gets its color from the brain's tens of billions of axons, each of which may make thousands of connections with other neurons.

Examining the cross-section slices he had taken from the brain, Markesbery noticed three small, pitted structures that resembled discolored cysts about the width of a pencil lead. These pits (lacunae) of dead tissue (infarcts) are the classic scars that most strokes leave behind. One of the lacunar infarcts was located in the white matter of the parietal lobe of the neocortex, a part of the brain involved in processing sensory information. The other two infarcts were in the deep regions of the brain's white matter, where damage can lead to problems ranging from personality changes to decreased intellectual acuity.

Lacunar infarcts often occur when small blood vessels become clogged with atherosclerotic plaque, a process that takes many years—which explains why the risk of stroke increases dramatically with advancing age. Although Markesbery could not determine with his naked eye whether atherosclerotic plaques had lined the walls of Sister Agnes' small blood vessels, they likely played an important role in the infarcts. He could see clear evidence of what he described as a "moderate degree" of atherosclerosis in the larger arteries at the base of the brain, the main entry point for the blood that nourishes it.

In addition to the three lacunar infarcts, Sister Agnes had had another type of stroke—one caused by the rupture of a blood vessel. Markesbery observed a tiny area of blood leakage, or hemorrhage, in the thalamus. Located deep within the brain, the thalamus partially serves as a signal relay station that helps turn thoughts into action. The hemorrhage likely damaged tissue there and further confounded communication through this network hub.

It was the microscopic examination that revealed the remaining damage. The plaques and tangles of Alzheimer's, it turned out, had riddled much of Sister Agnes' hippocampus and neocortex; indeed, the density and pattern of tangle deposition led Markesbery to rank her as a Braak stage VI, indicating the most severe level of Alzheimer's pathology.

So Sister Agnes had suffered from Alzheimer's disease, three lacunar infarcts, and a tiny hemorrhage. But how did these all fit together?

At the consensus conference we hold after every autopsy, Markesbery and I went back and forth over the pathological and clinical evidence. Plaques and tangles may have led to the degeneration of the gray matter in her neocortex that controlled Sister Agnes' thought processes, we reasoned. The small strokes in her white matter may then have added dramatically to her disability by disrupting the communication between her neocortex and other regions of the brain. In fact, the two kinds of damage may have had a synergistic effect.

To test our hypothesis—and to clarify how Alzheimer's and stroke might interact to produce dementia—we later decided to conduct a rigorous investigation of the Nun Study participants who had died by the end of 1995. To reduce variables caused by differences in education, we limited our analysis to sisters who had earned at least a bachelor's degree. In all, our study included 102 sisters, 45 of whom we had classified as demented based on our mental exams. What we found went beyond loosening the knot of confusion regarding how Alzheimer's disease and stroke interact—it challenged some of the most common diagnostic truisms.

Out of our entire sample, we found only one sister who had a textbook case of vascular dementia—that is, enough strokes in strategic locations to account for her dementia. She had essentially no evidence of Alzheimer's disease in her brain. Previous studies had asserted that vascular dementia accounts for up to half of the dementia seen in the elderly, second only to Alzheimer's disease. And of course this textbook wisdom became translated into diagnostic practice and treatment plans. This one sister's autopsy revealed only a few tangles in her hippocampus (she had a stage I rating on the Braak scale). But it also showed severe atherosclerotic plaques in her brain arteries and a massive infarction, spanning more than six inches, across crucial thinking areas of her brain.

As we reported in a 1997 paper published in the *Journal of the American Medical Association,* our autopsies showed that the small (lacunar) brain infarcts had a stunning link to dementia in the sisters—*but only if their brains also had enough plaques and tangles to meet our criteria for Alzheimer's disease.* Among the sisters with an "Alzheimer's brain," 93 percent had dementia if, like Sister Agnes, they also had at least one lacunar infarct in the deep white matter, the thalamus, or the neighboring basal ganglia (a collection of structures that control movement). In contrast, only 57 percent of the sisters who had an "Alzheimer's brain" but no strokes had dementia. Our data also suggested that sisters with evidence of a stroke required *fewer* tangles in the neocortex to show signs of dementia than if they had been stroke-free. We concluded that many sisters—in spite of having brain damage from Alzheimer's disease—avoided dementia because they had not suffered small strokes.

By 1999 we had analyzed the brains of 241 sisters, further clarifying the picture. Of these women, who ranged in age from 76 to 103 at death, we had determined that 118 had dementia. Autopsies of the demented participants revealed that 43 percent had Alzheimer's alone, 34 percent had a mixture of Alzheimer's and stroke, and only 2.5 percent had vascular dementia. (The remaining dementias were due to other causes.)

We always qualify our results by pointing out that the School Sisters of Notre Dame may not represent the population at large. Still, several other autopsy studies—including one conducted by Markesbery on Kentucky men and women—subsequently confirmed that vascular dementia is relatively rare. On the other hand, our research strongly suggests that small strokes serve as a trip switch in people who have significant numbers of Alzheimer's lesions, causing the symptoms of dementia to emerge. It also strongly suggests that stroke-free brains can compensate for Alzheimer's lesions to some extent and mute the symptoms of the disease.

—

This conclusion provides a real reason to hope. While we don't yet know how to prevent the plaques and tangles of Alzheimer's disease, we do have effective strategies for reducing the risk of stroke.

In my presentations around the country, I have now become a missionary for stroke prevention. High blood pressure causes more strokes than any other single cause. Antihypertension drugs, exercise, and a diet high in vegetables and fruits and low in fats all can help to lower the risk of stroke. If you are overweight, I tell people, even a moderate weight loss can bring down your blood pressure. If your cholesterol is high, take steps to bring it within normal range.

Weight loss also lowers your risk of diabetes. This is important because diabetes increases your risk for heart attack and stroke two to four times above that for people who do not have the disease. If you already have diabetes, it's important to work with your doctor and dietitian to maintain your blood sugar within the normal range.

Smoking is, of course, another key culprit in stroke. If you don't have enough reasons already to quit, add the possibility of dementia to your list.

I also urge people to learn the symptoms of stroke, which include numbness or weakness on one side of the body, confusion or trouble speaking, sudden vision problems, dizziness or loss of balance, or severe unexplained headache. It is important to seek medical care immediately if one is suspected. Even a ministroke (TIA) warrants medical attention. (The symptoms of a TIA may last only a few minutes, but they signal that a major stroke may be on the way.) Every minute that elapses after a stroke is critical, since drugs are available that can help slow down the cascade of events that eventually leads to brain damage. But these drugs work best within the first three hours. A stroke is a brain attack. It demands the same emergency attention as a heart attack. And that quick action can help to preserve precious mental functioning—even if the plaques and tangles of Alzheimer's have started to infiltrate the brain.

One evening after I had made such a presentation for the Alzheimer's Association, three generations of a family gathered around me—an elderly grandfather, two middle-aged couples, and their adolescent children. The patriarch was the first to speak. "Dr. Snowdon, several members of our family have had Alzheimer's. We'll go on any experimental drug regimen that you think would help us to avoid it."

I told him that the Alzheimer's Association was an excellent source of information about ongoing drug trials—among their many other services. But I reiterated that taking precautions to avoid stroke was a good defensive strategy that they could adopt immediately. One of the middle-aged men glanced at his wife. "Maybe I should quit smoking," he said. "The kids have been on my back about it anyway." To which I added a silent amen.

10

Our Daily Bread

Ever since the sisters heard about Dr. Snowdon's folate findings, they've been making a beeline for the salad bar.
—Sister Mary Aloysius Wieser

When Sister Mary Aloysius Wieser came to the Mankato motherhouse in 1941, the School Sisters of Notre Dame grew their own potatoes, beets, cabbage, cauliflower, broccoli, carrots, string beans, tomatoes, and peas. They had a large apple orchard, as well as a strawberry patch and huckleberry bushes. For meat, they raised their own cattle, pigs, and chickens, and they also had laying hens and milking cows. They baked all of their own breads.

"From 1941 until 1962, we had the same home service sister, Sister Verena Koppy, running the kitchen," Sister Mary Aloysius told me. Another home service sister, Sister Sabina Kierlin, for decades oversaw what Sister Mary Aloysius referred to as the convent's "victory gardens," the name given to vegetable plots during both world wars. (Both Sisters Verena and Sabina later joined the Nun Study.) The home service sisters were also responsible for the dawn-to-dusk work involved in canning and preserving the harvest every fall for consumption during the winter months. They did all this heavy work wearing their full habits covered with a long apron. Some sisters kept an older veil for such occasions.

The farm shut down slowly. First went the milking cows in the late 1940s; they had become more work than they were worth. When new houses went up at the base of Good Counsel Hill in the mid-1950s, the pigs and the beef cattle had to go. Until then, the sisters had stored the potatoes in the cattle barn, and the animals gave off enough heat to keep them from freezing during the winter. "We put lights in the barn to keep the potatoes warm, but then they sprouted early," Sister Mary Aloysius told me, laughing at the memory. The sisters stopped growing potatoes. Other vegetables soon went by the wayside, as did the chickens once the roof on their coop gave out.

By the late 1960s, most of the farming had stopped, and the Mankato motherhouse had become the retirement home for the province. In 1968, the doctors in the town of Mankato who cared for the sisters suggested that the convent hire a dietitian. So Sister Mary Aloysius, who then was teaching home economics at the Good Counsel Academy, went back to college at age forty-seven and earned a master's degree in nutrition. She returned to Mankato in 1971 as the dietitian. "I changed some of their cooking habits," she told me. The nutrient-laden liquids from cooking vegetables, which the sisters were pouring down the sink, would now be used in soups and gravies. She also added a variety of new vegetables and instituted a salad bar. And she began teaching the sisters about good nutrition and the value of various vitamins.

I was fascinated by the way these dietary changes on Good Counsel Hill—and similar changes at the other convents— seemed to sum up and make visible the larger shifts taking place in the United States as a whole. Many of the sisters in the early days came from farms and small communities that were largely self-sufficient in their food supply, and while we look back on this period with nostalgia, it is easy to forget the time-consuming, backbreaking work involved—not to mention the scarcity of fresh produce in the winter.

Sister Mary Aloysius was too young to participate in the Nun Study herself, but she became a valuable sister-scientist to add to our team. My first nutrition project at Mankato focused on the main difficulty of nutrition studies: determining what people eat and how that affects the nutrient levels in their bodies. When I raised chickens as a teenager, I could control exactly what was in their feed, but I couldn't control how much of it an individual chicken pecked up in a day. That was a minor problem compared to assessing human beings. The sisters at Mankato all ate food from the same kitchen, but the cafeteria-style meals still gave them considerable individual choice. And researchers have discovered that people are notoriously inaccurate in reporting what they have had to eat.

These problems were somewhat obscured in my earlier studies of the Lutherans and the Seventh-day Adventists. To be sure, we were relying on questionnaires, and hence on self-reporting. But the numbers were huge—eighteen thousand in the case of the Lutherans, more than twenty-five thousand for the Adventists—and our hope was that individual inaccuracies in reporting would be overwhelmed by the large sample size. Moreover, some of the crucial dietary differences among the participants were clearly defined. Among the Lutherans, we compared the health of men who drank alcohol with those who didn't. And since the Adventist church discourages meat consumption, our sample was neatly split between the approximately 50 percent who were lacto-ovo vegetarians (no meat, but some dairy products and eggs) and the 50 percent who ate some meat. The Mankato sisters ate a far more uniform diet.

Beyond the difficulty of determining intake is the difficulty of determining how the nutrients taken in are actually used by the body. People differ widely in how they metabolize food—as dieters lament, some people don't gain an ounce on the same meals that make others fat. As we age, the body's ability to digest food and absorb nutrients also changes. (For example, significant numbers of older people have difficulty absorbing vitamin B_{12}.) All of which adds to the complexity—and fascination—of nutrition studies.

I suggested to Sister Mary Aloysius that we first test whether our participants could accurately recall what—and how much—they ate during meals. We would weigh and measure the food on a standard-sized plate, and then videotape the sisters filling their plates in the cafeteria line. The following day we would ask them to detail what they had eaten at breakfast, lunch, and dinner the day before. Then we would compare their recollections with our more scientific measurements.

"We'll need to measure how much food they leave on their plates, too," I explained to Sister Mary Aloysius.

"I assure you that is not necessary," she replied. "You will find very little on their plates when they place them on the dishwashing cart. We do not waste. We were trained that way."

As I suspected, our video camera technique proved far more reliable than human memory. Sister Mary Aloysius' collaboration on this project resulted in her being named as coauthor on the first Nun Study paper on nutrition, which was published in 1990, when she was sixty-nine.

Since then, the Nun Study has contributed to some of the major nutrition findings—and controversies—of our time. As an epidemiologist steeped in nutrition studies, I of course dream of being able to demonstrate that certain foods or supplements protect the body, and especially the brain, from the effects of aging and Alzheimer's disease. The Nun Study has also evaluated possible links between toxins in the environment and Alzheimer's.

Although reports in the popular media, sometimes based on a single research paper, often suggest that "the solution" is at hand, the reality of science is different. We are repeatedly confronted with frustrating twists and turns in the evidence, and new research often undercuts previously accepted truths. This chapter is a journey through some of those twists and turns.

———

At the convent in Elm Grove, Wisconsin, I sat in the parlor one evening after supper chatting with Sister Mercedes Diederich, who had worked as a medical laboratory technician. Sister Mercedes followed the biological aspects of our study with particular interest. Our conversation on this occasion began with a question that I've heard many times in one form or another: "Should I only drink pop from bottles?" Sister Mercedes asked.

The idea that aluminum causes Alzheimer's disease dates back to 1965, when a study done on rabbits reported that injections of aluminum salts into their brains led to changes that resembled Alzheimer's disease in humans. Closer inspection later showed that the changes in rabbits were not the same as Alzheimer's pathology in human brains, but by then the "connection" between aluminum and Alzheimer's had been etched in the public's mind. Since then, the back-and-forth of this debate has made most researchers dizzy. The fear of aluminum toxicity has led many people not only to avoid soda in cans but to throw out all the aluminum pots and pans in their kitchen. Some popular publications have also advised people to stop using brands of baking powder, antiperspirant, and antacids that contain aluminum.

Of course, such fears are the mirror image of a greater underlying hope. If we could discover links between Alzheimer's pathology and toxins in the environment, we would have a potent weapon for combating the disease.

As I explained to Sister Mercedes, aluminum is the third most common metal in the earth's crust, and epidemiological studies in England, France, Norway, and Newfoundland have tied high aluminum concentrations in drinking water to Alzheimer's disease. Yet those studies used such gross measuring sticks with such broadly defined populations that they could not show a clear connection between aluminum and dementia. That would require autopsy studies.

As it happened, Bill Markesbery, in collaboration with University of Kentucky professor William Ehmann—a researcher known for detecting trace elements in moon rocks—produced some of the key autopsy data that argued against the hypothesis. In the early 1980s they published studies that found no correlation between Alzheimer's disease and the amount of aluminum in people's brains.

This is not to deny that aluminum has neurotoxic properties, which surface dramatically in patients with kidney failure who receive dialysis fluids containing very high levels of the metal. (In some cases, dialysis may result in 50 times the normal level of exposure.) This exposure seems to be associated with changes in tau, the stuff of the tangles of Alzheimer's disease. However, it still has not been shown that dialysis patients actually have more tangles in their brains than other people.

To date most Alzheimer's researchers, myself included, have been unconvinced by the evidence against aluminum. Given what we know today, I was comfortable telling Sister Mercedes that she should not worry about drinking soda from cans.

Concerns about another trace metal inspired a side journey for the Nun Study that none of us had anticipated. One day in

1992, Sister Mercedes, Dave Wekstein and I were strolling the hallways of the Elm Grove convent, when Wekstein noticed a door marked Dental Clinic. He insisted we go in, and when we did, we discovered that for the past three decades, the clinic had provided virtually all the dental care for more than 100 sisters at the convent. Wekstein seemed particularly animated and preoccupied by this news—although I couldn't tell why.

When we stepped back into the hallway, Wekstein explained. In 1990, the influential TV newsmagazine *60 Minutes* had broadcast a widely publicized report entitled, "Is There Poison in Your Mouth?" Some scientists had claimed that silver amalgam fillings, which are about 50 percent mercury, released mercury vapor when people chewed. This, they theorized, would accumulate in the body and cause Alzheimer's disease, among a host of other maladies.

The report had ignited an enormous controversy. The American Dental Association (ADA) dismissed the possibility that the minute amounts of mercury vapor released from fillings posed any health risk, noting that amalgam fillings had a safety record stretching back more than a century. The ADA took a particularly hard line against dentists who had recommended that patients remove silver fillings for health reasons, at which point some of the dentists sued their own organization for downplaying the risks.

Again, no one denied that mercury was a potent neurotoxin. This became apparent most tragically near Japan's Minamata Bay, where in the late 1950s and early 1960s more than two thousand people developed a crippling disorder of the central nervous system. After exhaustive epidemiological studies, ranging from analysis of the sludge in the bay to analysis of the hair of local fishermen and their families, scientists conclusively proved that the disease was caused by mercury contamination from local chemical plants.

The evidence against silver amalgam fillings rested on

much shakier ground. As the *60 Minutes* report detailed, people who had had their amalgam removed and replaced with non-amalgam fillings claimed to have been cured of long-standing illnesses ranging from arthritis to multiple sclerosis. Yet these anecdotal cases, as even the newsmagazine acknowledged, proved nothing.

More ominous was a 1990 study published by Markesbery and Ehmann that analyzed the levels of mercury and twelve other trace elements in autopsied brains. Brains from ten patients with Alzheimer's, it turned out, had significantly higher levels of mercury than the brains of twelve healthy controls, and the researchers cited dental amalgam as a possible source of the mercury. However, it was still an open question whether mercury accumulation was an *effect* of Alzheimer's disease or a cause.

Wekstein saw that the Elm Grove clinic might offer a unique source of data. When we returned to talk with the dentist, Sister Sara Jean Donegan, we learned that she was also a professor in the dental school at Marquette University. With her help, we designed a new investigation into the health effects of dental amalgam. We would compare the dental records of 129 sisters in the Nun Study with their scores on our cognitive tests. Would more fillings mean lower scores? Twenty-eight of the sisters had had all of their teeth removed and replaced with dentures—another interesting point of comparison. We supplemented the dental records by filming the mouths of the sisters with a small video camera. The videos were then examined by dentists at the University of Kentucky to confirm the actual number of fillings and the surface area of each.

Our analysis revealed no link between the amount of amalgam in the sisters' mouths and their function on eight different cognitive tests. When we adjusted our data for age and education, the disconnect between amalgam and mental status remained.

Consider two extremes from the study. When we did our battery of mental tests on Sister Albertine in 1991, she was eighty-six years old and had been wearing full dentures since 1945, when all her teeth were extracted. We also examined Sister Catherine, age seventy-eight, who had fourteen fillings—more than any of the other 128 sisters that we studied. Both sisters had master's degrees, so their level of education could not confound our results. Both also scored high on all of our mental function tests. Although they had a significant age difference on our first exam, Sister Catherine still had high scores on our mental tests when she was nearly eighty-two, which was her last assessment before her death. So Sister Catherine, despite having fillings in nearly half of her teeth, remained as cognitively fit as Sister Albertine, who had lived without her real teeth for the forty-six years before we tested her.

Our study, published in the *Journal of the American Dental Association*, made a persuasive case against the amalgam-Alzheimer's hypothesis. But it still did not address Markesbery and Ehmann's earlier findings about the levels of mercury in the brains of people with Alzheimer's.

Markesbery and Ehmann had looked at only ten Alzheimer's brains and twelve healthy controls, and they did not have access to the dental histories of these people. In addition, the techniques to detect small amounts of mercury had become much more sophisticated since their original study. So we launched a larger study combining Nun Study data with dental records and autopsy results from Markesbery's collection of brains donated by men and women from central Kentucky. Once again, we found no relationship between amalgam fillings and Alzheimer's disease. More important, we did not find any differences in mercury levels in the brains of Alzheimer's patients and the brains of the healthy controls—nor any relationship between the number of dental fillings and the level of mercury in the brain.

These findings challenged Markesbery's earlier conclusions, of course. "We're after the truth, whatever the data show," he said to me. "If we have to revise our thinking, then so be it. That's what science is about."

⟶

One of the first things I noticed when I started visiting the convents was how much mealtimes meant to the sisters. Other than the chapel, the dining hall is the one place where all the sisters are together, and especially for many of the retired sisters, meals are the major social occasions of the day. Certainly we Nun Study researchers did most of our bonding with the sisters at mealtimes. The air in the convent dining rooms buzzes with laughter and the lovely, distinctive pitch of elderly women chatting. Announcements are made about upcoming events, or about sisters who have fallen ill or recovered from sickness. At their tables, the sisters share news of former students and family members. The sports fans rejoice over or bemoan the fate of their favorite teams, while the politically inclined discuss the recent antics of the state governor or the president of the United States. This was a dimension of nutrition totally missing from my earlier research, and it turned out to have particular importance for the study of aging.

When I first went to Mankato, I observed that the dining area was divided into two sections. The healthy nuns assembled in one room and served themselves. The sisters in the assisted-living wing ate in another room just down the hall. Their food was brought to them, their medications were lined up at their places, and they could get help with cutting their meat or pouring their drinks. Only ten feet separated the two rooms, but moving between them felt like going from one world to another: one up and vigorous, the other quiet and disheartening—at least to me. Then several years ago the convent leaders decided to take a new approach. Both groups of sisters were reunited in one dining room. The results were wonderful to see. The able sisters quite naturally helped the less physically able to fill their food trays and get their drinks. The quiet sisters were drawn into conversation, and the sisters who had some cognitive problems seemed pulled toward the normal end of the spectrum.

While we didn't study whether this change made a difference in the sisters' nutritional status, I suspect it had a positive effect. Many studies have indicated that poor appetite and undernutrition are major problems among the very old. Our own Nun Study findings have shown that weight loss in the elderly is associated with a high risk of losing both mental function and physical abilities. Undernutrition may result from the problems I mentioned earlier—from changes in the way older bodies absorb or use nutrients. It may also result from the lack of easily available and varied food. (This was not a problem for the sisters, but it is crucial for many old people, who may not feel up to shopping and preparing food even when they have the money to buy it.) But depression, isolation, and lack of interest are often the critical factors.

The social importance of mealtimes was brought home to me one day in a conversation I had with one of our participants, Mother Georgianne Segner. Mother Georgianne, a Texan from the Dallas province, had been general superior of the worldwide congregation during a most difficult time. She assumed office in 1968, when hundreds of School Sisters of Notre Dame in Soviet-bloc countries were isolated and living under severe restrictions. At considerable personal risk, she repeatedly visited Eastern Europe, often under police surveillance, in order to offer them support. After she returned to Dallas in 1977, she became pastoral minister in a nursing home that later began serving young AIDS patients. At age seventy-seven, she became involved in a program to bring hot meals to AIDS patients living in a nearby apartment building and encouraged other sisters to join her. As Mother Georgianne explained, the sisters would not only prepare and deliver the food, but also stay to visit. Healthy nutrition required warm conversation as well as hot meals, she said.

Again and again at the end of public lectures, I am asked about substances that are supposed to "save the brain"—vitamin E, ginkgo biloba, selenium, melatonin, choline, and L-acetylcarnitine, among others. In some cases I feel there is enough evidence to justify cautious experimentation. Just as often, however, I have to respond, "We don't know yet."

It is at moments such as these that I recall Mother Georgianne's work and my memories of the mealtime buzz at the convents. What I know for sure is that nutrition for healthy aging is not just about eating certain foods or downing a certain number of milligrams of a prescribed number of vitamins each day. It also depends on where we eat, whom we eat with, and whether the meal nourishes our heart, mind, and soul as well as our body.

—

About the time Sister Mary Aloysius returned to Mankato as the convent's dietitian, vitamins were becoming big news. I had learned in middle school that they prevented obscure diseases like scurvy and rickets, but by the early 1970s, my college professors were saying that they played a much larger role in health—and specifically that they might offer protection against aging and disease. Vitamin E seemed to slow the aging of the skin, and possibly of other parts of the body. Nobel prize-winning chemist Linus Pauling was proposing megadoses of vitamin C as a cure for the common cold—not to mention diseases ranging from cancer to schizophrenia. More convincing evidence was accumulating that fruits and vegetables offered protection against heart disease, stroke, and some cancers. In a landmark 1981 article in *Nature*, British scientist Richard Peto argued that the orange pigment beta carotene was the key anti-cancer component of vegetables and fruits—which raised the status of ordinary foods such as carrots, winter squash, and cantaloupe to that of health powerhouses.

What vitamins C and E and beta carotene have in common—together with many other substances—is that they are all antioxidants. They protect the body from oxidative stress— the wear and tear we incur simply by being alive. The same process that causes iron to rust and plastic to get brittle and crack with age also affects the tissues and organs of our bodies. Every breath we take carries oxygen into our cells, where metabolism produces unstable oxygen molecules, called free radicals, that react with other nearby molecules—often in destructive ways. Oxidation is one of the central unifying theories of aging and disease. Among other effects, oxidation causes the skin to lose flexibility and start to wrinkle; it promotes the accumulation of atherosclerotic plaque on artery walls; in the joints, it increases the inflammation of arthritis; it damages the lens and retina of the eye; and it increases the risk of some cancers.

Markesbery and other scientists have proposed that oxidation plays a major role in Alzheimer's disease. Compared to healthy controls, brain tissue from Alzheimer's patients shows higher levels of oxidation. Amyloid, the ingredient of the plaques, also appears to generate free radicals that add to the damage done to neurons. And tissue damage in turn creates more free radicals—setting off a destructive cascade of events that can lead to the atrophy and death of brain tissue.

The body limits the damage by producing its own substances to absorb free radicals, but we can assist this mopping-up process by increasing our consumption of antioxidant foods or vitamins. So the persuasive theory goes. Yet after a quarter century of studies, the picture is far less clear than scientists expected it to be.

In 1993, I began a new collaboration with Christine Tully, a geriatrician at the University of Kentucky who was interested in nutrition. Tully wanted to measure certain micronutrient levels in the blood to see whether we could discover any links to the mental status of the sisters, and she and I went to Mankato to explain our project to the Nun Study participants there. The sisters took to her right away; they seemed to appreciate that as a woman physician, she had made her way in a male-dominated field. By the end of our presentation, all ninety-five of the participants had agreed to fast overnight and then donate a blood sample.

Part of each sample was sent to Myron Gross, a nutritional biochemist who was a friend from my days at the University of Minnesota. Gross had been studying the role of antioxidants in heart disease and cancer and was delighted to extend his research into aging. We agreed that he would measure the plasma level of vitamin E and a general class of antioxidants called carotenoids. (Carotenoids are pigments, such as beta carotene, that protect plants from damage by the sun's ultraviolet rays.)

This would be one of the first human studies on antioxidants and aging, so when the first results came in, we were primed for a discovery. To our disappointment, however, none of the five carotenoids—including beta carotene—showed any relationship to cognitive function or Alzheimer's. To our even greater disappointment, neither did vitamin E. (By then, vitamin E was being touted as a neuroprotective agent, particularly because of its antioxidant properties.)

One item in our data set, however, really caught our eye. A carotenoid called lycopene showed a strong correlation to *physical* function in our Mankato sisters. The sisters with the lowest lycopene levels in their blood more frequently needed help performing self-care tasks such as bathing, dressing, standing, toileting, and feeding.

Lycopene is a red pigment found in a small number of plants, including tomatoes, guavas, watermelon, and pink grapefruit. There is no equivalent substance produced in the human body, so we have to get it from these few foods. In addition, there is evidence that lycopene is best absorbed when it is consumed with some fat. In other words, a lycopene pill might not have the same effect as lycopene in a tomato-based spaghetti sauce. And unlike some vitamins, which are damaged by cooking, lycopene is actually more available from cooked tomatoes than from fresh ones. (From this perspective, even pizza takes on a new, healthful aspect if you skip the pepperoni and extra cheese.)

In 1999, three years after we published the results of our first antioxidant study in the *Journal of Gerontology*, Myron Gross and I returned to the blood samples to see if we could find a relationship between longevity and antioxidant levels. Once again lycopene seemed to have a strong link to survival. Six and a half years after the sisters had donated their blood samples, we found that 70 percent of those with high blood levels of lycopene were still alive, compared to only 13 percent of the sisters with low levels. (None of the eighteen other nutritional markers in our study had significant associations with survival.)

As potentially exciting as this seemed, neither of our studies permitted us to do more than note the association of lycopene with health. We could not show that it actually *prevented* disability or death. We had not monitored the blood of the sisters over time, so we could not determine whether the low lycopene levels actually occurred before the appearance of disability. It's equally possible that the high oxidative stress caused by ill health and disability had "eaten up" much of the available lycopene in the sisters' blood. That same oxidative stress may also have placed them at higher risk of dying. In this case, lycopene's potent antioxidant properties might make it a barometer of health rather than a cause.

Since other studies conducted during the past ten years suggest that lycopene may offer protection against heart disease and cancer of the breast, lung, bladder, and prostate, Myron Gross and I remain optimistic about its potential benefits.

Meanwhile, vitamin E had gotten a boost from an Alzheimer's study that was published in 1997. The "big" finding from this elaborate clinical trial was that eighty-five moderately demented Alzheimer's patients given vitamin E supplements remained healthier than a control group that took a dummy pill, or placebo. However, the devil was in the details. After two years of observation, vitamin E supplementation appeared only to delay institutionalization of the Alzheimer's patients. It had no clear relationship to mental or physical function or to survival.

The editorial that ran with the article in the *New England Journal of Medicine* carried the downbeat title, "Treatment of Alzheimer's Disease—Searching for a Breakthrough, Settling for Less," and it commented that the results were "encouraging but should be viewed cautiously." Nevertheless, the report was widely touted in the media. And many physicians responded by prescribing vitamin E, sometimes in combination with vitamin C, to their patients with Alzheimer's.

That same year saw the publication of a paper in the *Journal of the American Medical Association (JAMA)* on the herbal remedy ginkgo biloba. The leaves of the gingko tree contain a number of powerful antioxidants, and a standardized, patented extract of the leaves is widely prescribed in France and Germany to improve blood flow. The *JAMA* article reported on a clinical trial that seemed to confirm earlier reports of ginkgo's modest effectiveness in stabilizing early Alzheimer's disease and in some cases even improving cognitive function. However, this trial was criticized for incomplete data collection, and the editors of *JAMA* came under fire for even publishing an article about such an unconventional substance.

Nonetheless, to my mind, the ginkgo findings were more convincing than those from the vitamin E trial. Yet because ginkgo is considered "alternative medicine" in the United States, relatively few doctors recommend it to their patients. That, of course, does not prevent widespread popular use, since the standardized extract is available without a prescription. However, both patients and doctors lose in this situation—patients because dosages and side effects may not be monitored, and doctors because they do not gain clinical experience with a potentially useful supplement.

Inconclusive or inconsistent findings such as those for vitamin E and ginkgo are pretty much par for the course. I was struck by this when I attended a seminar that Myron Gross gave at the University of Kentucky early in 2001. Part of his presentation was a review of recent major studies on the relationship of antioxidants to heart disease and stroke, and after a few examples, my head began to swim with names and numbers. The CHAOS study of more than 2,000 heart attack patients reported that vitamin E might prevent a second heart attack. The NHANES study of more than 11,000 people reported that vitamin C might prevent a *first* heart attack. The Nurses Health Study (which included 87,245 women) found that vitamin E, but not vitamin C, might provide protection against heart disease, while a study of nearly 5,000 people in Rotterdam reported no effects for vitamin C or vitamin E but a protective effect for beta carotene. And the HOPE study of 9,000 patients with a history of cardiovascular disease failed to live up to its name—it found vitamin E no better than a placebo in preventing a recurrence of either heart disease or stroke.

These were well-designed studies that, overall, involved more than a hundred thousand people. The human studies of antioxidants and Alzheimer's disease, which are based on only hundreds of patients, have produced equally equivocal results. What message, then, can we take from so much effort on the part of researchers? Scientists such as Gross and Markesbery still believe that oxidation is vitally important in the major chronic diseases. And after weighing results from laboratory, animal, and human studies, they still believe that antioxidants such as vitamin E hold great promise in reducing the risk of stroke, heart disease, and Alzheimer's disease.

—

Nine years into the Nun Study, we finally found a nutrient that appeared to stave off the brain-damaging effects of Alzheimer's disease in the sisters. This research is dear to my heart not only because of our results, but also because of the way it illuminates my own field, epidemiology. The great insights in epidemiology often come into focus slowly, like a jigsaw puzzle with hundreds of pieces. In this case, the first pieces were laid in place two centuries ago, and the picture includes such disparate elements—including nuns and pregnant women—that we hardly would have expected to fit them together at all.

An eighteenth-century Dutch midwife named Catherina Schrader was the first to link poor nutrition in mothers to neurological damage in their infants. Like a pioneering epidemiologist, Schrader kept meticulous records on thirty-one hundred births over five decades. Six of those babies had the severe brain and spinal cord deformities that we now call neural tube defects, and all of those births occurred among poor women after periods of severe crop failure.

It was not until 1965 that neural tube defects were conclusively linked to a deficiency in folic acid, or folate, a B vitamin found in abundance in dark green leafy vegetables, such as spinach and kale, and in beans, nuts, citrus fruits, and liver. That year, researchers in Liverpool, England, published a landmark paper on pregnancy outcomes in the British medical journal *The Lancet.* They documented that 66 percent of the mothers in their study who gave birth to infants with brain and spinal cord malformations were deficient in folic acid—in contrast to only 17 percent of the mothers who had normal babies.

This paper was followed by a major nutritional trial conducted by the influential British Medical Research Council and completed in 1991. Supplements of folic acid were given to pregnant women who earlier had given birth to babies with neural tube defects. The supplements reduced by 70 percent a woman's risk of having another baby with similar problems.

These amazing results spurred a massive public health campaign to ensure that all pregnant women take folic acid supplements. In a further protective measure, the U.S. Food and Drug Administration mandated in 1996 that folic acid be added to grain products such as breakfast cereals, enriched breads, and pastas.

But what does this have to do with the cognitive abilities of elderly nuns? Two years after the *Lancet* study linking low folic acid levels to birth defects, a report in another medical journal suggested that folic acid deficiencies might also be linked to dementia. This report, and several others that followed, were based on anecdotal evidence from case reports of demented patients. More provocatively, a 1977 report on sixteen older adults suggested that folic acid deficiency might lead to brain atrophy—the shrinkage of the brain seen in Alzheimer's disease.

For nearly twenty years, however, this small but important study went virtually unnoticed. (It's impossible to know why, but research on nutrition and disease had gone under something of a cloud after the excitement of the early '70s. I attribute this partly to the medical and scientific backlash created by the exaggerated claims of Pauling and others.) Then, in 1996, I received a call from an editor at the *Journal of the American Medical Association,* asking whether I would serve as one of the outside reviewers of a paper that tied low folic acid levels to Alzheimer's. When I received the paper, I was impressed by what I found.

Researchers at the Oxford University Project to Investigate Memory and Ageing (the OPTIMA study) had reported that low blood levels of folic acid may be linked to a high risk of Alzheimer's disease, as well as to a greater degree of brain atrophy. Their paper immediately made me think of our Mankato blood samples. Although we had used them up in our micronutrient study, we had created a large database that I could easily search. We not only had folic acid measurements, by then we also had brain autopsy reports on thirty of the sisters who had died. A quick analysis raised my eyebrows high: Our data fit beautifully with the observations of the Oxford group.

I found myself in a most peculiar bind. I badly wanted to speak with the Oxford researchers to discuss the possibility of submitting a manuscript that might run in conjunction with their own paper, which raised two problems. Reviewers ethically cannot take an idea from the paper under consideration and use it to get a leg up on the competition—or, worse still, to scoop the paper itself. Scientific journals also typically insist that reviewers remain anonymous to allow colleagues to freely critique each other without fear of reprisals or recriminations. But because of this unusual situation, I received permission from the editors at the *Journal of the American Medical Associa-*

tion to contact the Oxford researchers, and we soon began to compare data.

Our Nun Study folate research focused on the thirty Mankato sisters who had died since contributing their blood sample. When we correlated the results of their autopsies with the folic acid levels in their blood, we found a striking connection: The higher the folic acid level in the blood, the lower the chance of brain atrophy.

Since Alzheimer's can be viewed as a "brain wasting" disease, it is reasonable to think that folic acid deficiency could move the process of atrophy into high gear. The Oxford study had also suggested a biological mechanism behind this link: Folic acid's relationship to Alzheimer's disease might be due to another substance in the blood called homocysteine. This made things even more interesting.

Homocysteine is essential to the body's functioning, but it can also participate in the process leading to atherosclerotic plaque. High levels of homocysteine are now considered one of the primary risk factors for heart disease and stroke. One of the most crucial roles of folic acid in the body is to join with vitamin B_{12} in breaking down homocysteine into its useful form. If the body lacks enough of these vitamins, the homocysteine accumulates, with far-reaching consequences.

The Nun Study has underscored the connection between vascular diseases and Alzheimer's. But laboratory evidence also suggests that homocysteine itself may damage and kill brain cells, thus speeding the atrophy of the Alzheimer's brain. This would explain why brain atrophy is related to both low folic acid and high homocysteine levels in the blood.

Several other small studies of folate have since replicated the findings of both the Nun Study and the Oxford OPTIMA study. Definitive evidence of the protective effects of folic acid in Alzheimer's may come in a few years, with the completion of a large-scale randomized clinical trial sponsored by the National Institutes of Health. Even though dashed hopes are an occupational hazard for those who do nutrition studies, I am particularly optimistic about folic acid.

When I tell men about our findings, they respond with moderate interest. But women truly light up, especially if they've had a child. As soon as they were pregnant—or even before they conceived—their doctor urged them to increase their folic acid intake. Now it appears that the substance that has such dramatic impact at the beginning of life may guard life's end as well.

—

If we could lock several thousand people away for a couple of decades, precisely control their diet, and then observe the health consequences, we might have the clear answers we all want about nutrition and Alzheimer's disease. But of course we can't do that—and, in the meantime, we have to eat.

When I asked Myron Gross what he, as a nutritional biochemist, recommended, he emphasized that vitamins and other nutrients are potent biological substances that can affect different people very differently, depending on the dose and on the person's genetic makeup, her medical history, and the medications she is taking. For example, very high doses of vitamin E can cause gastrointestinal and bleeding problems, a particular hazard for the elderly. While most people don't need their doctor's permission to take vitamins and other food supplements, it is essential to tell your doctor what you are taking.

Gross told me that his own nutritional program is quite simple: He eats a diet high in fruits and vegetables, takes a standard multivitamin every day, and takes an additional 200 IU of vitamin E on alternate days. Because he has a family history of heart disease, he also takes an aspirin about twice a week.

Neurologist Bill Markesbery recommends that his patients in the early stages of Alzheimer's disease take considerably higher doses of vitamin E, vitamin C, and folic acid. He also recommends a trial of a prescription anti-inflammatory drug, such as celecoxib (brand name Celebrex), which is less likely to cause stomach ulcers and bleeding than aspirin or other common anti-inflammatory drugs. These drugs may help to reduce the brain-damaging effects of the inflammatory process in Alzheimer's disease. (Epidemiological studies have shown that people taking anti-inflammatory medication for rheumatoid arthritis have a significantly lower risk of Alzheimer's.) The intake of high doses of vitamins or anti-inflammatory drugs should be under the watchful eye of a physician, because they can have serious side effects.

As an epidemiologist wanting to preserve my own long-term health, I view nutrition much the way I view the stock market. I avoid putting all my money into a couple of big-name stocks, and I diversify my portfolio with mutual funds. In the same way, I avoid getting on the bandwagon of a few currently "hot" nutrients. I take a standard balanced multivitamin each day, one that provides the full daily value for nutrients such as vitamin E (30 IU), vitamin C (60 mg), and folic acid (400 mcg). On alternate days I take two pills instead of one. This gives me a nice margin—about 50 percent higher intake of a broad range of nutrients than is usually recommended.

The most important component of my health investment portfolio is eating a wide variety of fresh fruits and vegetables. More and more promising nutrients are being discovered in plants—well beyond the standard vitamins and minerals. Some of these are new antioxidants, while some are other phytochemicals (*phyto* means "plant") that have a wide range of health-promoting effects. As with so many things that affect our health, it now appears that these nutrients work synergistically.

So while scientists bob and weave through the thickets of dietary research, it may be that heaping our plates at the salad bar—like the one Sister Mary Aloysius was so proud of—is our best nutritional strategy for warding off aging and Alzheimer's disease.

11

Up and Grateful

Even with three philosophy exams from Father Ooghe each year
and the bugbear of ten hours of practice teaching, I am still
enthusiastic about every day, every hour, spent within the halls
of Notre Dame College.

—Sister Genevieve Kunkel

One week before Christmas 2000 and two weeks before her ninetieth birthday, Sister Genevieve Kunkel marveled at her well-being. "I have two good traits," she told me. "I am alert and I am vertical."

Sister Genevieve was prone to understatement. Sister Genevieve, who prefers to wear a veil with regular clothing, was one of the liveliest characters I had met at Villa Assumpta, a convent near Baltimore that houses about a hundred School Sisters of Notre Dame. Not only was this short and sprightly former teacher of English in fine physical health, but during the preceding year she had read a best-selling novel (*The Pilot's Wife*), the memoirs of Father George Dunne (*King's Pawn*), and nearly every issue of the Sunday *New York Times.* She still corresponded with many of the students she had taught at elementary and high schools in Maryland and Massachusetts. "My girls are grandmothers now!" she boasted. One, Sister

Genevieve excitedly noted, recently sent her a box of books that included a copy of *Harry Potter and the Sorcerer's Stone.* "I can't wait to read it," she told me.

Sister Genevieve then launched into a story about a sister who came to Villa Assumpta five years ago. This sister, who had suffered from a lifetime of depression, said, "Sister Gen, you're always so up. What's your secret?"

"I didn't know what to say," Sister Genevieve confided to me, "but I thought she deserved an answer, so I told her, 'Maybe it's because I've always been with the young.' "

Baptized Genevieve Louise, this eldest of nine children helped care for her siblings. As she told it, even driving her brothers and sisters to school had an upside. "For my sixteenth birthday, Papa gave me a new Chevy sedan, the latest model with a roll-up windshield," she recalled fondly. "Then Papa took my little Chevy and I drove the family's seven-passenger Marmon to Notre Dame every day." Throughout her four years at the College of Notre Dame of Maryland, Sister Genevieve continued to taxi her younger siblings around, staying closely involved with their lives. After graduating with a bachelor's degree in 1932, she entered the School Sisters of Notre Dame as a postulant. Three days later she found herself teaching at St. Mary's High School in southern Maryland. And for the rest of her career, educating young people—from grade school through college—remained her life and her love.

"Why shouldn't I be up?" Sister Genevieve asked me, returning to the question again. "Up and grateful." Showing her penchant for one-liners, which she often used in her classrooms, she then offered this nugget of wisdom: "Give your attitude some altitude!"

Over the years I have met countless elderly sisters who similarly have delighted me with their sunny, chipper personalities. At first I attributed this largely to the sisters' spiritual training and to their lives of purpose and service. But Sister Genevieve's history revealed to us that the sisters' spiritual formation was only part of the story—and helped lead the Nun Study to a most astonishing discovery.

—

Comparisons between individual sisters sometimes guide us in our investigations, helping us to decide what would be most fruitful to study in larger groups. The more closely two sisters' lives overlap and yet have different outcomes, the more readily we can identify the factors that led to their unique fates. The lives of Sister Genevieve and a sister I will call Penelope overlap more closely than most.

They were born in Baltimore two years apart, but they were in the same grade at school because Sister Penelope, the older of the two, did not start until she was seven. (Her mother wanted to extend her daughter's childhood play.) Both their fathers operated successful family businesses—Sister Genevieve's owned and operated a piano store, and Sister Penelope's sold building supplies—and both girls grew up in the comforts of the upper middle class. Both were the eldest children of large families. Both earned their B.A.'s at the College of Notre Dame of Maryland and entered the candidature in the Baltimore convent in the early 1930s. From the mid 1930s through the 1950s they taught high school in Massachusetts, and earned master's degrees in their spare time. They later worked in supervisory positions at various schools run by the School Sisters of Notre Dame around the United States. Their lives intersected again more than sixty years after they joined the congregation, when Sister Penelope, who had begun to experience physical problems (or, as she told a friend, "the shady side of the so-called sunny years"), moved into Villa Assumpta.

However, a striking and crucial difference between them emerged in 1999, when we started a new analysis of the autobiographies that they had written as novices.

—

During our first study of the autobiographies in the early 1990s, my collaborator Lydia Greiner and I had been astonished by their individuality, especially since the writers were responding to a standard assignment. We were especially interested in the difference between the writers we called "listers" and the "high-fidelity" writers, the ones who wrote with sensuous detail and vivid feeling. We had actually tried to code the autobiographies for their emotional qualities at that time, but we set this data aside when idea density proved to have such a clear relationship to Alzheimer's.

In 1999 I started working with two colleagues at the University of Kentucky's Center on Aging who reignited my interest in the autobiographies: Deborah Danner and Wallace Friesen. Danner is a psychologist who specializes in emotion; she had done fascinating research based on her observations at a local Alzheimer's support program called Helping Hand. Friesen had done pioneering investigations into the relationship between emotion and physiology. He was the coauthor of a famous study, published in *Science* in 1983, which showed that simply instructing people to show various emotions on their faces greatly changed their heart rates. His later research had confirmed that happiness, anger, surprise, fear, disgust, sadness, and other basic emotions have specific impacts on the autonomic nervous system, which controls such involuntary functions as heart rate, blood pressure, immune response, and digestion.

Other researchers have been following this link, and the relationship between stressful emotions and heart disease is by now well established. When we feel threatened, whether emotionally or physically, the famed fight-or-flight response floods our body with chemicals that drive up our blood pressure, among many other physical effects. When the threat is past, the body usually returns to normal. But some people live in a war zone—either literally or because they have a heightened response even to minor threats. When the fight-or-flight response is strong enough or persistent enough, the body can't compensate. That is why habitual anger and hostility are known risk factors for heart disease, and depression is a risk factor for both heart disease and stroke. (The "broken heart" of bereavement has turned out to be almost literally true as well. Many elderly spouses outlive their partners by only a few months.)

Because I was aware of these links, I wanted to find a way to test whether emotional expression in the sisters was related to longevity. Related research had been ongoing at the famous Mayo Clinic in Rochester, Minnesota, resulting in a study published early in 2000. The Mayo researchers had followed 839 patients who had been classified as optimists or pessimists on standardized personality tests given in the early 1960s. Thirty years later, significantly more optimists were still alive. The researchers duly noted that "the exact nature of interactions between the mind and body evades explanation." But they offered intriguing possibilities. Maybe optimists were less likely to develop depression. Maybe pessimists did not seek medical care as promptly. Or there could be biological mechanisms at work, such as more robust immune systems in optimists; one 1998 study provocatively suggests that positive emotions might actually "undo" the cardiovascular stress triggered by negative emotions.

Findings such as these led us to return to one of the original goals of the Nun Study: to explore the factors contributing to longevity. Could the sisters' autobiographies, written when they were healthy young women, predict how long they would live?

——

For our study, Danner, Friesen, and I assembled handwritten autobiographies from 180 sisters who had taken their vows in the Milwaukee and Baltimore provinces. (These provinces had divided into two additional provinces during the 1950s and 1960s, so our sample also included sisters living in the Chicago and Wilton motherhouses.) Working with a new team of coders, we identified every word that reflected an emotional experience. The coders classified these words as positive, negative, or neutral.

This is tricky territory for research because of the dangers of subjective judgment. The coders worked independently of one another, and the protocol was strict. Only when their assessments coincided and were checked by a third coder were they entered into our database. And once again the coding was blind—no one knew the health status of the sister concerned.

In the end, the coders read some 90,000 words and determined that only 1,598 of them related to emotional experiences. They ultimately classified 84 percent of these words as expressing positive experiences (happiness, love, hope, gratefulness, contentment), 14 percent as negative (sadness, fear, disinterest, suffering, shame, disgust), and 1 percent as neutral (surprise).

First, consider Sister Penelope's two-page autobiography, which contains a total of eight sentences:

> I was born on October 7, 1909, the eldest of eight children—five girls and three boys. In my seventh year, I entered St. Elizabeth's Parochial School. My High School

studies were pursued at Notre Dame of Maryland and my collegiate courses at Notre Dame College and Johns Hopkins University Summer School. As regards my vocation to the religious life, it was undoubtedly influenced by my contact with Notre Dame Sisters during the sixteen years I spent in Notre Dame schools. The School Retreat given in February 1932 at the College was the first occasion of my asking advice on the matter and definitely determining to answer the call of our Savior. On May 26, 1933, my application for admission was filed at the Motherhouse on Aisquith Street and on September 8th, I entered. My candidate year was spent in the Motherhouse, teaching Mathematics and English Literature at Notre Dame Institute. With God's grace, I intend to do my best for our Order, for the spread of religion and for my personal sanctification.

Although Sister Penelope's autobiography rated high in idea density—the measurement so important to our previous study—it reads like a neatly written business letter. The coders concluded that it expressed no emotion whatsoever.

—

Sister Genevieve's autobiography went on for five pages, and her forty-one sentences kept the coders busy.

When I was first told that I saw the light of day on a Tuesday noon, there automatically ran through my mind the old nursery rhyme pretending to predict one's fate by making it depend on the day of the week on which one was born. It goes something like this

"Monday's child is fair of face;
Tuesday's child is full of grace—"
Now, I don't want to feign that I had dreamed of being a

nun from the age of reason but it at least was a good en-
couragement and something to strive for as an ideal.

Interestingly, this lovely opening to Sister Genevieve's autobiography was coded for only one emotion, and it was a negative one at that. The phrase in the last sentence that begins
"don't want to feign," the coders decided, showed disinterest.
Of course, most readers might protest that "good encouragement" or striving for an ideal qualify as positive ideas. But the
study imposed a rigorous discipline: to code only words directly indicating emotions.

As Sister Genevieve's autobiography continues, the positive
soon starts to outweigh the negative.

> *I remember little of my baby days and what I do I have had*
> *to take on hearsay. From all accounts I was perfectly nor-*
> *mal with regard to mischief and, being the first of my fond*
> *parents' offspring, might have become their spoiled darling*
> *had God not blessed them as the years went by with eight*
> *others to share their love and care.*

The coders scored two positive emotions here, keyed to the
words *fond* and *love.*

> *How thankful I am that He selected me to be one of a large*
> *family for now I realize there is no compensation for those*
> *who miss its joys and sorrows.*

This single sentence expressed two positive emotions
(*thankful* showed gratefulness, and *joys* evinced happiness)
and one negative (*sorrows* was sadness).

Sister Genevieve's autobiography then recounts her elementary school days, in which she describes herself from the
start of kindergarten as a happy, interested pupil.

One incident of those days stands out most vividly. My teacher, Sister Pamphilia, rewarded me with a dainty white prayerbook for saying the alphabet backwards. I was proud of it and I don't think I could perform that feat today!

She notes her first communion with particular joy.

Young though I was, I can recall with sweetest memories that day of days when, as Sister Stilla had instilled into us, our Guardian Angels were especially vigilant and loved us more than ever before.

School to her was "a quest for knowledge," and she was especially thrilled to enter college.

The third Wednesday of September, 1928, I was enrolled as a Freshman at the College and then followed the happiest days of my scholastic career. Hard work coupled with loyal friends and jolly times kept away all monotony. Even with three philosophy exams from Father Ooghe each year and the bugbear of ten hours of practice teaching, I am still enthusiastic about every day, every hour, spent within the halls of Notre Dame College. Time, when one is contented, flies by swiftly and before I could fathom it, the first day of June of '32 found me with a sheepskin in my hand and a tear in my eye. It is hard to go forth from the protecting wings of such an alma mater; to go forth from the loving care of those who trust in one to a world that is eager to play upon the frailties of its newcomers.

Happiness, contentment, eagerness, love, and enthusiasm spill from these sentences, which, according to the coders, expressed positive emotions seven separate times.

Yet Sister Genevieve was no Pollyanna. As if anticipating our reaction so many years later, she wrote:

> *As I reread the foregoing paragraph, I realize that one might easily think the learning process went on without its tilts and tumbles. I beg to correct that notion, for always the day dawned not fair and often were the times when doubt gripped my heart and clouded every hope and project.*

Sister Genevieve went on to write an earnest, soul-searching attempt to explain why she entered the School Sisters of Notre Dame.

> *I must admit that I never pictured myself as a religious. In fact, so unaware was I of it that as a sophomore I was fully determined to become a private secretary and study law in between. That is one of the funniest ideas, I think, that I ever entertained. Probably, all unknowingly, the seeds of vocation were first sown when my eldest brother and special pal left at sixteen to become a Jesuit. Our visits with him each Thanksgiving and summer made a deep impression and turned my mind to the great question of "what doth it profit?" His growth in physical health and spiritual peace made me reflect and it is to his example of courage and perseverance that I gratefully attribute my own following of Christ's call. Of course the annual retreats at school, especially those of my last college years, prepared the way but his ready sacrifice of all that was near and dear gave me something concrete to ponder over and imitate.*

As did most of the novices, Sister Genevieve closed her autobiography on a spiritual note, but hers again stands out for its lyricism and, to borrow a phrase from her, great joy.

And now, that I am really a Postulant and with the great joy of Reception less than five weeks away, I pray Jesus to make me less unworthy to become His Spouse and may Mother Theresa, from her high place in heaven, look down upon me and plead with her Heavenly King to enrich my soul with graces which will help me to be a faithful daughter of her own School Sisters of Notre Dame.

As the Proverbs in the Old Testament declare, "A merry heart doeth good like a medicine, but a broken spirit drieth the bones."

In the autobiographies of Sister Genevieve, Sister Penelope, and 178 other School Sisters of Notre Dame, written when they were an average age of twenty-two years old, positive emotional content strongly predicted who would live the longest lives. This is a most extraordinary finding: A writing sample from early adult life offered a powerful clue as to who would be alive more than six decades later.

Astonished by our own results, we analyzed the data from several angles, carefully adjusting statistically for age, education levels, and linguistic ability. Each time, we arrived at the same conclusion, which is most simply appreciated by breaking the sisters into four groups based on the ranking of their expression of positive emotions. In the group that had used the fewest positive-emotion sentences, the average age of death was 86.6 years old. Sister Penelope in fact lived longer than the average for her group. She died of a sudden heart attack at age 89.

The average age of death went up to 86.8 for the second group, 90.0 for the third, and 93.5 for the sisters who, like Sister Genevieve, flooded their autobiographies with positive emotions. From the low to the high end of the scale, positive emotions accounted for a survival difference of 6.9 years.

Another fascinating way to view these results is to look at the mortality in each of these four groups at different points in time. When we did this analysis, we found that the sisters who scored the lowest number of positive-emotion sentences had twice the risk of death at any age when compared to those who were in the highest group.

There is an important caveat here: Sister Penelope lived to be 89, a long life by anyone's measure. Clearly, the lack of positive emotions at a young age does not foretell an early death. In addition, Sister Penelope was hardly a negative person: A friend who spoke at her wake recalled that it was characteristic of Sister Penelope "to find life good, exceedingly good."

The real question, however, is subtly—but critically—different: Does a positive outlook early in life contribute to longevity? Our data suggest that the answer is yes.

In the world of science, you are lucky if a study is accepted for publication within several months to a year after it is submitted to a peer-reviewed journal. Our manuscript on positive emotions and longevity was provisionally accepted by the *Journal of Personality and Social Psychology* in two and a half weeks— a new record for the Nun Study, and a sign of the provocative nature of our findings.

Over a celebratory lunch at the faculty club, Danner, Friesen, and I began to muse about some of the larger implications of what we had discovered. As scientists addressing other professionals, we are limited to writing about what we can test. But as human beings, we look beyond our data to the unanswered questions and speculate about how our discoveries impact our daily lives.

In her studies of Alzheimer's patients, Deborah Danner had found that memories connected with strong emotions were often retained even when the patient had appeared to have lost contact with the outside world. Before visiting a patient, she would brief herself on the high points of that person's life—the events that had brought them the most happiness. Then, during a videotaped interview, she would talk with them about those memories. Even family members were often astonished at the outcome of these visits: Withdrawn patients who had stopped speaking altogether sometimes became animated and even responded verbally to her questions.

Danner recalled telephoning the wife of a severely impaired patient to ask permission to talk with him about his feelings. The couple had been married for fifty-five years, and the wife told her outright, "You can come, honey, but he doesn't know enough to feel." Her husband had been bedridden for several years and rarely uttered a word. When Danner was alone with the patient, she recalled the celebration the couple had had for their fortieth wedding anniversary. She saw the man smile. Reassured, she went on, scanning his face for nonverbal signs of comprehension. Imagine the wife's surprise when she suddenly heard her husband's voice from the other room. One of the things he said to Danner: "I don't talk because no one listens anymore."

My luncheon discussion with Danner and Friesen then took off in a different direction: the question of *why* some people seem naturally positive and expressive, while others tend to remain neutral—or even dour. It is now widely accepted by psychologists that this is not simply a matter of upbringing, although childhood experiences have a major—and sometimes decisive—influence on how we develop. Babies clearly come into the world with an inborn temperament. From their earliest days, their responses to their environment tend to cluster somewhere on a spectrum: highly sensitive, reactive, and hard to comfort, on one end; resilient, steady, and easy to please, on the other. (Friesen, with three children of his own, readily endorsed this view.) How much of this difference contributes to what we would later call negative or positive personality? What can we do to help a "difficult" child learn to handle stress in a more balanced, positive way? And how much can adults modify their own reactions to stress—possibly in response to data such as ours?

I told Danner and Friesen that my work with them had made me more aware of my own stress responses and that I now made a conscious effort to regain my physiological balance quickly after an upset. Sometimes I have to express the negative feelings strongly in order to resolve them; I've learned that this can be a good thing. Sometimes I'm able to put them into perspective simply by shifting my mind to more positive aspects of my life and remembering the things I am most grateful for. In either case, I try not to stay stuck in negativity. My goal is to return my body to its normal, healthier state as soon as possible.

Over our long lunch, we also considered how we might go beyond the limitations of our study. One problem was that we had too little data to adequately assess the role that negative emotions played in survival. The sisters had expressed few negative emotions in their autobiographies. This may simply have reflected the reality that these young women were at an exciting juncture in their lives: They were about to take their vows, and many soon would leave the provincial house for their first teaching or domestic assignment. And of course they were aware that their superiors would read what they had written.

Not only did this make it difficult to understand how negativity impacts longevity, but it also obscured our attempts to figure out the physiological mechanisms responsible for the good or poor health of a sister. Did the key difference lie in whether the emotions expressed were positive or negative? Or was it the difference between richness of emotional expression—both positive *and* negative—and suppression of emotion? Popular wisdom and research have, at various times, lined up behind both positions. We simply don't have the answer.

Our initial emotions study did not attempt to probe the connections between emotional expression and Alzheimer's. We now plan to compare what we have learned from the sisters' autobiographies with the mental and physical exams we give them. And as more of the Nun Study participants die, we will incorporate the information that we learn by examining their brains. I am confident of this much: We are in for many surprises.

We know from the outset that Alzheimer's and longevity often have a harsh relationship: The longer you live, the more likely you are to develop the symptoms of the disease. But we also know that approximately 55 percent of people who live to be eighty-five or older do *not* develop symptomatic Alzheimer's disease. Ideally, then, our work will help to understand the factors that allow the Sister Genevieves of the world both to live long lives and to retain their mental faculties to the end.

As medical advances and improved living conditions allow ever more people to survive for nine decades (and beyond), the quality of life versus its quantity presents a staggering challenge to the so-called oldest old—and to those who care for them. The more experience I have with the older sisters, the more I realize how few of us hope simply to survive. We want to retain our ability to reason, to remember, to express our thoughts, to read a new novel or the newspaper. We want, as much as possible, to remain independent of others when it comes to moving about, dressing, eating, and using a bathroom. We want to be spared the suffering caused by chronic illnesses. We want to live in communities with people we love and people who love us. In short, we want to have what Sister Genevieve has—including, odd as it might sound for a woman who is now ninety years old, a future filled with hope.

12

The Hundred-Year Marathon

*I don't want to say we rejoiced at putting her to rest, but it
wasn't a crying funeral. She had gone to God after 102 years,
and we were sending her off.*
—Sister Mary Busson on the funeral of
Sister Mary Mark Woltering

Villa Assumpta is the provincial house for the School
Sisters of Notre Dame in Baltimore, and on the day of
my visit there in the spring of 1991, it was also the
home of the oldest person I had ever met.

At age ninety-eight, Sister Mary was an unforgettable presence. Her full black-and-white habit was topped by a long-
beaked green tennis visor, which, as I later learned, she wore
to shade her eyes from glare. And she was tiny: about four and
a half feet tall and all of eighty-five pounds. She had a big,
openmouthed smile, remarkably smooth skin, and eyes that
radiated a playful suggestion of peace and joy.

Sister Louis Marie Koesters, who introduced us, had prom-
ised me that Sister Mary was "quite something." But I didn't
discover just how "something" until Sister Mary and I had
chatted for a while. After we got acquainted, I told her a little

about how I had started the Nun Study, and then I got down to business. Despite her pleasant conversation, I assumed that this very old and apparently frail sister must be a bit out of touch. So I began with the simplest of questions to assess her mental function.

"Sister," I asked, "who is the president?"

"Why, that would be George Bush," she politely replied.

"What's today's date?" I asked.

"April twenty-fifth, 1991," she said, giving me a quizzical look—perhaps she was wondering about *my* mental state.

"Where did you live ten years ago?"

"Well, let's see. Right here. I retired in 1976."

"Where did you live forty years ago?"

Sister Mary did some math out loud, explaining that she had taught at St. Peter's in Philadelphia from 1959 to 1976 and at Pittsburgh's Most Holy Name for three years before that—which brought her back to St. Patrick's in Cumberland, Maryland, where she had been assigned to teach eighth grade in 1949.

Sister Mary could even tell me the name of her first mother superior in 1910, the year she was received into the novitiate.

My head spinning, I thanked Sister Mary and said my good-byes. I still could not quite believe that at her age she could accurately recall such fine details from so long ago. So I went to the convent's archives and checked her records. They confirmed that she had been correct about every last fact.

Sister Mary had been a teacher for more than sixty years, and on that day she taught me an indelible lesson about what scientists call the "oldest old." Yes, time had taken a toll on her body, and she suffered from a long list of health problems that included arthritis, heart disease, and anemia. But from our first conversation, I recognized that her mind was remarkably intact. During the following two years—during which she cele-brated her one hundredth birthday—my fascination grew as we carefully analyzed her abilities and simultaneously explored her long history. Time, I concluded, surely causes wear and tear on the body: Almost everyone's hearing is compromised by one hundred, and no one gets that far with 20/20 vision. The mind, however, ages by a unique calendar. And the more centenarians I would meet, the more convinced I would become of this truth.

The Nun Study was not specifically designed to study centenarians. We look, instead, to the work of researchers such as my friend Thomas Perls, a geriatrician at Harvard Medical School. His project, the New England Centenarian Study, is described in his book *Living to 100,* which he co-wrote with neuropsychologist Margery Hutter Silver. Perls and Silver explore this new social phenomenon in great detail. Centenarians have become so common, they note, that Hallmark now makes special birthday cards for people who make it to the magical age of one hundred. Indeed, the U.S. Census Bureau projects that the number of centenarians in the United States will jump from fewer than thirty thousand in 1990—80 percent of whom were women—to more than eight hundred thousand by 2050. Centenarians are actually the fastest-growing age group in the country.

As of the beginning of 2001, a total of eighteen of the sisters in the Nun Study had celebrated their one-hundredth birthdays. It remains a mystery to me how these women have lived a century or longer and, in several cases, remained as sharp as Sister Mary. But as I learned the details about their pasts, as we gathered information about their mental and physical capabilities, as I came to know them as individuals, and as we analyzed their genes and their brains—thirteen now have died—clues to their longevity have begun to emerge.

Two of these factors cannot be scientifically tested by the Nun Study data, and yet after fifteen years of working with the sisters, I believe strongly in their importance. The first is the deep spirituality that these women share. My sense is that profound faith, like a positive outlook, buffers the sorrows and tragedies that all of us experience. Evidence is now starting to accumulate from other studies that prayer and contemplation have a positive influence on long-term health and may even speed the healing process. We do not need a study to affirm their importance to the quality of life.

The power of community is the second factor that the Nun Study is not designed to measure. However, evidence on this score is accumulating from other research, including a famous long-term study, published in 1979, that followed residents of Alameda County, California. It has now been convincingly documented that marriage, membership in churches, clubs, or other social groups, and regular contact with family and friends all reduce the risk of death from the major killers, coronary heart disease and stroke.

For more than fifteen years now, I have witnessed how the School Sisters of Notre Dame benefit from their ever-present network of support and love. The community not only stimulates their minds, celebrates their accomplishments, and shares their aspirations, but also encourages their silences, intimately understands their defeats, and nurtures them when their bodies fail them. From the day they enter the convent, they are members of a congregation that existed long before they were born. On the day they are laid to rest, they are celebrated by a community that will endure long after they are gone. How many of us are held so securely throughout life?

This is not to say that centenarians such as Sister Mary are more spiritual or more involved in the community than sisters who die at a younger age. Rather, I believe these factors help to shift the distribution of age at death in the entire congregation. The risk of death in any given year after age sixty-five is about 25 percent lower for the School Sisters of Notre Dame than it is for the general population of women in the United States. This means that the sisters live dramatically longer lives than their lay counterparts. The centenarians simply represent the leading edge of this phenomenon.

⟋

The day that Sister Mary turned one hundred, September 15, 1992, I happened to be attending a conference on successful aging at the National Institutes of Health in Bethesda, Maryland. As Villa Assumpta is only an hour's drive away, I decided to stop by that afternoon and offer Sister Mary my best wishes in person.

One of the speakers at the morning conference had presented a study that investigated the effects of different kinds of support on physical function in the elderly. The researcher's data suggested that *emotional* support—including simply listening and talking in an affirmative way—could slow the development of disabilities. On the other hand, it appeared that offering unnecessary *physical* support—such as dressing an older person who can do it herself, or providing a wheelchair when she can manage with a walker—actually increased the incidence of disability.

When I arrived at Villa Assumpta later that afternoon, these thoughts were swirling through my head. Sister Mary proved to be in a somewhat irritable mood, tired of dealing with the media folks who had come out to report on her hundredth birthday. I took her wheelchair handles and started to move her away from the hubbub, but then it struck me that this was the very sort of assistance that might actually do her more harm than good. I'd seen her wheel herself, so I wondered who I was doing this for. Myself or her? But then I thought, Cut her some slack! She's a hundred years old! I wheeled her away.

Sister Mary did not need any theories to help her age successfully.

Born in 1892, when Benjamin Harrison was president of the United States and Victoria was queen of England, Sister Mary was the eldest of eleven children. She grew up in a working-class neighborhood in Philadelphia, where her father, a German immigrant, was a foreman in a hat factory. When she was thirteen her mother died in childbirth. In 1907, shortly after she graduated from St. Boniface elementary school and before she turned fifteen, Sister Mary became a postulant with the School Sisters of Notre Dame in Baltimore. She was soon dispatched to the same Philadelphia elementary school to teach the first grade. By the time she was received into the novitiate in 1910, when she was all of seventeen, she had taught in elementary schools in Cumberland, Maryland, and Rochester, New York.

Sister Mary made her first vows in 1912. In 1935, her superiors allowed her to make her very first home visit, to see her father on his deathbed. He died the next day, and she was granted permission to return to Philadelphia the following week to attend his funeral.

Sister Mary went on to teach the seventh and eighth grades for forty-two years. At age seventy-seven she cut back her hours and became a part-time teacher and teacher's aide. At eighty-four she finally retired from teaching. But if you asked her, Sister Mary would not admit to being retired. "I only retire at night," she would say.

When Sister Mary moved to the assisted-living wing in 1983, she kept going. She helped the sisters who had not fared as well as she, clearing their dishes and reminding them to take their medications. She also began to use a map or a globe during her prayers, dedicating a separate day to each continent. She avidly read newspapers and books, magnifying glass in hand and her trademark green visor over her veil. The other sisters loved to tell her that she looked like a bookie.

In 1990 she decided to donate her body to the Anatomy Board of Maryland. In letters she wrote to her family, she declared it "one of the happiest days of my life." One year later, when we gave our formal presentation about brain donation to the Baltimore sisters, Sister Mary was right up front by the lectern, and I could see her nodding even before I finished speaking.

In our formal Nun Study assessment shortly after she turned 101, Sister Mary performed remarkably well. She correctly identified nine of the fifteen line drawings in the Boston Naming test and eight of the twelve real objects in the Object Naming test. Her score was 9 out of a possible 12 on the Constructional Praxis test, which required her to copy geometric shapes of increasing complexity. Not only were these scores above average, but they were especially notable given her somewhat impaired vision. Her short-term memory was also above average for the study: In the Delayed Word Recall test, she remembered five of ten words, and she identified eight out of ten in the Word Recognition test. And her score of 27 out of 30 on the Mini-Mental State Exam matched her astounding performance during my first visit in 1991.

The nurses at Villa Assumpta told us that she had not had any noticeable mental changes over the preceding decade, although they did affectionately report that during the past few years she had stopped "bossing the other sisters around."

By early June of the following year, as Sister Mary approached her 102nd birthday, nursing reports indicated that she still had no problems remembering a short list of items, grasping situations and explanations, or recalling recent events. However, she had become "quieter" and "less energetic."

At 6:45 P.M. on June 13, 1994, Sister Mary passed away from

colon cancer. At her death, she weighed only seventy pounds. Her green visor was on display at the wake held in her honor. As the sisters reminisced about their good friend, one told this story: "I remember her telling me that one day she had wondered out loud to her doctor if perhaps he was giving her medicine to keep her alive when after all her desire was to be with Jesus. To which the doctor replied: 'Sister, it's not my medicine that's keeping you alive. It's your attitude!' "

When we autopsied Sister Mary's brain, another question confronted us: Why hadn't she shown any symptoms of Alzheimer's? Her brain weighed a mere 870 grams. At that time we had autopsied the brains of 117 other sisters, and only five of the brains weighed less. We also found that she had nearly three times the average number of tangles in her hippocampus seen in the other sisters. Intriguingly, however, she had very few tangles in her neocortex, and she had no infarcts that marked a stroke; this may explain why she was spared the symptoms of Alzheimer's disease.

Sister Mary added significantly to the small but growing evidence that the risk of Alzheimer's does not steadily increase in the oldest of the old. As Perls reported in 1998, the six brain autopsies he did as part of his New England Centenarian Study (only 20 percent of his participants agreed to donate their brains) showed not a single case of definitive Alzheimer's disease. In fact, it appears that the people who make it through their nineties without developing Alzheimer's are actually at a lower risk than people in their eighties. As Perls puts it in *Living to 100,* "the older you get, the healthier you've been."

Think of the nineties like the Boston Marathon's Heartbreak Hill, which appears at about mile twenty-one of the twenty-six-mile race. A man traditionally stands there with a sign that reads It's All Downhill from Here. Almost everyone who makes it past that point finishes the race. Sister Mary, then, was one of those ultrafit marathoners who cruise across the finish line. And over the years since her death, the Nun Study has discovered other champions of aging.

—

At the end of a hallway in the Mankato motherhouse, between the nurse's station and the elevator, hangs a bulletin board that I make it a point to visit each time I am at the convent. Pinned to the board is a handwritten list of the sisters who are ninety or older.

Regina ~~99~~ ~~100~~ 101†	Hedwigis ~~93~~ ~~94~~ 95†
Matthia ~~99~~ ~~100~~ 101	Mary Stanislaus ~~93~~ ~~94~~ 95
Augustine ~~99~~ ~~100~~ 101	Rita ~~93~~ ~~94~~ 95
Esther ~~98~~ ~~99~~ 100	Estelle ~~93~~ ~~94~~ 95†
Verena ~~98~~ ~~99~~ 100	Anne Mary ~~93~~ ~~94~~ 95†
Borgia ~~98~~ ~~99~~ 100	DeSales ~~92~~ ~~93~~ 94
Marcella ~~98~~ ~~99~~ 100	Alonza ~~92~~ ~~93~~ 94†
Wuna ~~98~~ ~~99~~ 100†	Agneta ~~92~~ ~~93~~ 94
Mary Clemens ~~98~~ ~~99~~ 100	Cornelia ~~91~~ ~~92~~ 93†
Edith ~~96~~ ~~97~~ 98†	Mary Cyril ~~91~~ ~~92~~ 93
Louise ~~96~~ ~~97~~ 98†	Marcelline ~~91~~ ~~92~~ 93†
Rose ~~95~~ ~~96~~ 97†	Mechtild ~~91~~ ~~92~~ 93
Candida ~~94~~ ~~95~~ 96†	Jane Frances ~~91~~ ~~92~~ 93
Camilla ~~94~~ ~~95~~ 96†	Sabina ~~91~~ ~~92~~ 93
Margaret ~~94~~ ~~95~~ 96†	Mary Clement ~~91~~ ~~92~~ 93
Remigia ~~94~~ ~~95~~ 96	Mary Ann ~~90~~ ~~91~~ 92†
Dorothea ~~93~~ ~~94~~ 95†	Clarice ~~90~~ ~~91~~ 92
Alphonsetta ~~93~~ ~~94~~ 95†	Cleta ~~90~~ ~~91~~ 92†
Hyacinth ~~93~~ ~~94~~ 95†	Berenice ~~90~~ ~~91~~ 92
Mary Jane ~~90~~ 91†	Terese 90
Anna ~~90~~ 91†	Amalia 90†
Florence ~~90~~ 91	Francetta 90

Blandina ~~90~~ 91   Germaine 90†

Almeda ~~90~~ 91   Lioba 90

Loretta ~~90~~ 91†

The list strikes me as both regal and sacred, its power accentuated by those wonderful antique names: Matthia, Borgia, Remigia, Agneta, Cleta.

At each birthday past ninety, a line is put through a sister's age and her new age is added. Small crosses indicate those who have died. The list above was posted on November 25, 1995, the day Sister Marcella turned one hundred. For the next nine months, the Mankato convent would enjoy the presence of seven sisters who had lived a century or longer. They came to be called the Magnificent Seven.

Not all of the Magnificent Seven enjoyed good health, but time had spared two of my closest Mankato friends, Sisters Esther Boor and Matthia Gores.

I first contacted Sister Esther in 1986, as the pilot study was taking shape at Mankato. At the time Sister Esther was teaching at a religious education center in Montana. She was ninety-two and had earned her master's degree in theology at age seventy-one. "I'm too busy to be in a study about old people," she told us. Of course, mentally fit people in their nineties were exactly whom we wanted to study, but we never pressure a sister to participate in our project, and I forgot about Sister Esther for a time.

At ninety-seven Sister Esther decided to retire and return to the Mankato motherhouse, promptly joining the Nun Study— and wowing all of us.

Sister Esther had entered Mankato as a postulant in 1912, the year the convent was built. The eldest of eight daughters, she had been taught by School Sisters of Notre Dame since the first grade. After Mass one day when she was still very young, she told her parents, "If I were a boy, I'd be a priest."

Her father, a tailor and dry cleaner, didn't miss a beat. "You're a girl," he answered. "You can be a nun." On the evening before her first communion, her parents had her stay with the sisters "to avoid all distractions and keep the silence," as she explained in her autobiography. "It was during this time that the thought of entering the religious life became firm in my mind."

Back on Mankato's Good Counsel Hill eighty years after she first arrived, Sister Esther began helping with the care of ailing sisters, working at the reception desk, pedaling an exercise bike each weekday for ten minutes, and painting figurines (a favorite is Santa on a John Deere tractor) in the convent's Ceramic Haven. She also filled her days doing crossword puzzles, reading mysteries, writing letters to relatives, and, during baseball season, closely following the fate of her Minnesota Twins. She used a spiffy-looking walker, replete with hand brake and a basket, to get around, although she would insist to me that she really did not need it. She was so short that her feet did not reach the ground when she sat in a chair, so she strategically placed footstools about the convent, including one in the chapel. To alleviate pain from her arthritis, she received regular hot wax treatments for her hands. "It loosens my hands so my writing isn't so bad," she confided.

Sister Esther started greeting me with the same line each time I visited Mankato: "I'm still alive."

At the end of my visit, I offered her a stock goodbye that became part of the joke: "Don't go dying on me."

Sister Matthia was also born in 1894, and she had become a postulant in Milwaukee in 1910, before the School Sisters of Notre Dame had even acquired the fifty acres on Good Counsel Hill. She moved to Mankato in 1913 and then—after teaching elementary school in Wisconsin, Minnesota, and Washington State for sixty-two years—she retired to Good Counsel Hill in 1971, when she was seventy-seven.

Shortly after I met Sister Matthia, she invited me to her room for a chat. "Let me show you my students," she said. She then opened an old notebook in which she had written down the names of all 4,378 of the girls and boys she had taught, together with their grades, schools, and ages.

"Every day I say a prayer for all of them," she explained. If she learned that a former student had died, she placed a cross by the name and said extra prayers.

As the Nun Study received ever more media attention, Sister Matthia became something of a celebrity. At 103 she appeared in *Time* magazine. Later that same year, in November 1997, *National Geographic* ran a photo of her long-fingered, heavily wrinkled hands knitting a pair of mittens. "I don't like that photo," she told me. "It makes me look old." Her hands looked beautiful to me.

Sister Matthia knitted one pair of mittens each day, donating her handiwork to local charities. At the suggestion of Sister Bernardia, her biological sister (who died in 1987 at 95), she kept track of the number of mittens she had made: more than fifteen hundred pairs. One day that fall she asked me what color I liked, and by evening a pair of thick dark green mittens was waiting outside my door in a brown paper bag. Sister Matthia told me that she had learned to knit and crochet in the first grade, when she was six, so that by the time she knitted my mittens, she had ninety-seven years of experience. They hang on my office bulletin board to this day, a small reminder of the way the centenarians have reshaped the way I think about time, old age, and living well.

Sister Matthia has also changed the way I think about memory. The Nun Study tests represent our best efforts to quantify memory and how it changes as we age. But our scientific tools cannot grasp memory's true richness and depth—the qualities evoked by Sister Matthia's unusually lengthy autobiographical writings.

From an autobiography she appears to have written in the early 1970s, shortly after she retired, I learned that Sister Matthia had honed her deft storytelling skills the same way she became a master knitter: with routine, dedication, and decades of practice. "The first days of each year, I agreed with my class that I would tell them a story ten minutes before dismissal if all behaved well during the day," she wrote. "Any pupil who failed to meet the requirements could not hear the story and would be assigned special work in a different room. This proved to be a keen incentive and most pupils met the challenge. . . . The stories were like a magic wand." So as not to repeat herself, she recorded in a little blue book the date and title of each story told.

The most eye-opening autobiography Sister Matthia gave me vividly re-created what it meant to be a School Sister of Notre Dame in the 1910s. True to Sister Matthia's meticulousness, she had made two drafts of this autobiography. She wrote the first twenty-one-page draft shortly after her diamond jubilee in 1975—the celebration to mark the sixtieth anniversary of her first vows—when she was eighty-one. I presume she was not pleased with the quality of her handwriting or the level of detail, because she then wrote a forty-six-page version in a perfect Palmer cursive. Reading it was like opening a time capsule.

Sister Matthia and eighteen other postulants in the Milwaukee province normally would have been received into the novitiate in 1912, but the mother superior convinced her class to wait another year so that they could have their ceremony at the new Mankato chapel.

In March of 1913, when the nineteen postulants moved into the new convent on Good Counsel Hill, they hauled their own furniture up three flights of stairs. "Men to help were very few," she remarked. In addition to a fix-it man, they had a gardener, seventy-two-year-old Mr. Wind—"an old man" in her estimation, which he certainly was by the standards of 1913. "We postulants helped him carry the many stones found in the ground into the ravine or gully down the Hill," she wrote. "It was great!"

As part of their preparation, a chaplain instructed them—in German, which they all spoke—about what was expected of a School Sister of Notre Dame. " 'A Religious,' he said, 'lives more securely, falls more rarely, rises more quickly, and dies more peacefully.' . . . He warned us not to hang our heart on any other person, but Christ," Sister Matthia recalled. "And not to get too free with any person of either sex. God is a jealous lover and wants our whole heart."

The postulants could invite as many relatives as they wanted to their Reception Day, but the novitiate marked the beginning of a much stricter and more austere life. Sister Matthia had an early experience with the vow of poverty. In honor of the ceremony, her mother had knitted her an exquisite pair of wristlets "made from real fine, black silk thread," she noted. "I showed them to Mother Isidore [the mother superior], and she said: 'They are too nice for you. Give them to me. I will sell them for a good price to a fancy, rich lady, then we can use the money to help pay for our new buildings here.' " On Reception Day, her mother asked why she wasn't wearing them. "I told her: 'You see, Mother, today it is rather warm, and I am wearing a common pair.' I did not have the heart to tell her I could not keep them, because I did not want to hurt her, as she had long and carefully worked to knit them for me. I was glad she never inquired about them again."

Following the ceremony, the novices were not permitted to eat with their relatives, but instead had their first meal with the professed sisters and visiting Church dignitaries. Sister

Matthia continues her account with an undercurrent of humor. "After we said the table prayers together, all the Sisters knelt and kissed the floor—now, we just newly received Novices were just aghast at the scene," she wrote. While they were eating, she noticed a visiting sister superior kiss her bread. "I thought: My, my, that must be a particular, fancy Sister, who smells her bread before eating it—as if it were moldy." Then it occurred to her that perhaps eating moldy bread was part of being a nun. "Well, if that is all we have, then we must also be real satisfied with that," she told herself. "I'm sure it won't kill us, otherwise, not so many Sisters would live to be so old."

During the next year, the novices could speak with their classmates only during evening recreation. Sister Matthia could not even speak with her biological sister, who lived in another section of the convent for part of the year. "I think this seclusion was really a fine test of obedience, self-denial and penance," she wrote. The novices became grateful for the smallest exceptions, such as the visits with other sisters that were allowed on Christmas and Easter and the few mealtimes when speaking was allowed. "The 11 days in the year that we were permitted to talk at the table were really great events," she recalled.

Each day began at 5 A.M., when a bell rang to signal that the novices had twenty-three minutes to dress and be in place at the chapel for morning prayers. They then worked on the grounds, milking the cows, feeding the pigs and sheep, and helping Mr. Wind in the garden. They also received twice-weekly lessons from Mother Isidore. One day she walked the novices to the brow of Good Counsel Hill and showed them six thorn bushes that she had brought from Jerusalem as slips; when they took their first vows, she told them, they would receive crowns made from these very thorn bushes. She then pointed to the Mankato homes below. "She said if we knew how many tears are shed there in one day and night, we would be surprised how much sorrow we find in one city alone," recalled Sister Matthia. Mother Isidore also stressed that the sisters must be willing to bear pain and discomfort without complaining.

Sister Matthia also gave me an obituary that she wrote for herself in 1996, when she was 102. "I am a little slow in getting my thoughts," she confessed. She recounted how two of her biological sisters became School Sisters of Notre Dame and one of her brothers a priest; including her first cousins, her family had eleven sisters and five priests. "Now regarding my *long* living, it seems to be a special reward from God," she wrote.

In May 1998 Sister Gabriel Mary administered what would be our last mental exam of Sister Matthia. The exam included a request for a short autobiography, which Sister Matthia wrote neatly, without difficulty. "God help me, please, to reach Heaven safely after I die," she wrote in closing. Late on the afternoon of December 14, 1998, a few weeks shy of her 105th birthday, Sister Matthia asked a sister who was at her bedside to notify her relatives that she was dying. The oldest living School Sister of Notre Dame then received communion and passed away forty-five minutes later.

At her wake, the crown of thorns she had received when she took her vows—which had been carefully stored for eighty-three years—was pinned to the inside of her coffin. Nearby was the three-inch crucifix she had also received at that 1915 ceremony. Made from metal with a black wood inlay surrounding the body of Christ, it had been polished smooth by years of prayer. Her sisters did not bury it with her. Instead it was given to one of the province's young novices, who keeps the crucifix on a table in her room and prays next to it every day. It has become part of Sister Matthia's legacy to a new generation.

On December 9, 2000, the Nun Study hosted a conference at the University of Kentucky for forty scientists who study Alzheimer's disease the same way we do, by following groups of people over many years. The title of my talk was "Getting to Very Old Age, and What's It Like When You Get There." I showed a four-panel photograph of the autopsied brain of Sister Borgia Leuther, the Mankato sister who had made the handmade cards that my mother so loved. From every angle, in every slice, her brain appeared normal. Her Braak staging was a zero, indicating that she had virtually no signs of Alzheimer's pathology. She had no evidence of strokes, either. When I announced that Sister Borgia had died at 103, I heard many ohs, ahs, and wows from the audience.

Sister Borgia's brain bowled us over, too. "It's one of the most amazing brains I've ever seen," Bill Markesbery said. "It looks like it came from a sixty-five-year-old."

As of the beginning of 2001, we have autopsied the brains of nine centenarians in the Nun Study, and here is what we know: The risk of stroke increases dramatically with age and peaks in the late nineties. Half of the people who die between ninety-five and ninety-nine have brain infarcts—evidence of stroke. In the over-one-hundred group, only 22 percent of the brains have infarcts. The older brains appear less damaged.

This holds true, too, when we look at the progression of Alzheimer's pathology. It appears to increase with age, hit a plateau, and then decline. In the Nun Study, we find that 40 percent of the sisters who die between eighty-five and eighty-nine have severe Alzheimer's pathology—Braak stages V and VI. But only 22 percent of the sisters who die at one hundred or older have this level of Alzheimer's pathology in their brains.

Our data suggest that whatever causes Alzheimer's disease

may dramatically slow its assault by about age ninety-five. That is a terrifically encouraging message for baby boomers. More and more people are living to one hundred because of scientific advances such as pasteurization, vaccines, antibiotics, and improved nutrition. What will be the average lifespan of the baby boomers who have enjoyed these advantages their entire lives? Is ninety-five so far-fetched? And forty or fifty years from now, what will the brains of ninety-five-year-olds look like? Will the scientific and medical advances enjoyed by the boomers also result in healthier, more functional brains? We are entering truly unknown territory, but I am more and more hopeful about what we will find there.

The Nun Study, of course, is all about exploring the unknown, and we intend to remain on that frontier. We want to clarify the dividing line between Alzheimer's and what are now called mild cognitive impairments so that we can evaluate more precisely where someone falls on the spectrum of disease at a given point in time. This may help us find ways to prevent the conversion of mild cognitive impairment into full-blown Alzheimer's disease.

We also are attempting to develop more sophisticated methods for evaluating the living brain. By collating all the images from our brain MRIs with Markesbery's autopsy data, we are developing a computer model that will help us predict the equivalent of a living person's Braak stage. This will enable us to more accurately identify people at high risk.

Soon we will also start screening hundreds of genes to search out those related to longevity and successful aging. We plan to look more closely at the many biological sisters we have in our study. We also hope to extend our research on emotion and to investigate the role of personality, which is one factor on which the sisters differ widely from person to person.

I am often asked whether we will end the Nun Study when the last sister dies. Hardly. We will mine this data for decades to come—and I suspect that others will comb through it long after Markesbery and I are gone. As Markesbery has often said to me, "This is a once-in-a-lifetime study." Opportunities to track over time a clearly defined and uniform population such as the School Sisters of Notre Dame are becoming ever more rare in the modern world. This is one motion picture that likely can never be filmed again.

Right now, I believe that we will be collecting data for another twenty years. As of the start of 2001, 295 of the original 678 participants were still alive. The average age of the participants was eighty-nine; the youngest was eighty-four. So far, more than three hundred brains from the deceased participants have been studied under Markesbery's microscope. And as we continue to develop new hypotheses, Markesbery goes back to inspect many of the first brains collected, all of which are being carefully preserved for future study.

—

As 1999 drew to a close, the sense of expectancy and suspense that the entire world shared was heightened for the centenarians in the Nun Study. If they made it past December 31, not only would they participate in the turning of the millennium and the great Jubilee Year proclaimed by the Pope, but they would be able to say that they had lived in three centuries.

Of the Mankato Magnificent Seven, two sisters were still living: Sister Esther Boor and Sister Mary Clemens Slater were both 104. Sister Mary Clemens had stepped down after many years coordinating the Santa Anonymous program, which provided Christmas gifts for hundreds of poor children. In

Chatawa, Sister Mary Mark Woltering of the Dallas province, a lifelong kindergarten teacher known for her kindness, had already celebrated her 101st birthday. In Wilton, Sister Cordis Impler, age 101, had only recently stopped reading the *New York Times*—her eyes, not her mind, had failed her. And in Milwaukee, Sister Maurice Pfeiffer, who was known as a jigsaw puzzle fan, still had her good sense of humor and her sweet tooth at age 102. The Nun Study also had two living "century babies," born in 1900. Sisters Karla Conder in Chicago and Clementa Abel in Milwaukee were preparing to cross the 100-year mark.

So the record stood on December 29, 1999, when about a hundred sisters, friends, and relatives gathered in the dining hall of the Mankato motherhouse to celebrate Sister Esther Boor's 105th birthday. Red and green helium balloons that said "Let's Celebrate!" floated above each table. Sister Esther, a corsage pinned to her habit and hearing aids in both ears, held court at the front of the room.

Two of the guests of honor were Sister Esther's twin sisters, age eighty-nine, who wore identical Christmas sweaters and windbreakers. "From the time they were born, I slept with them every night," Sister Esther bragged.

"They love you around here," a sister told her as yet another camera flashed.

"I can tell," she said.

A sister playing an accordion led a rousing "Happy Birthday," and another sister took Sister Esther's arms and began dancing around her, the queen sitting on her throne. Sister Esther then clapped her hands to "You Are My Sunshine," and the crowd sang along: "Please don't take my sunshine away."

As the party wore on, the provincial leader kneeled down to speak with Sister Esther. "Happy birthday to you," she said. "How's it going?"

"Pretty good," said Sister Esther.

"Are you tired?"

"I feel two hundred and five-ish," she admitted.

But then she brightened. "I've had so much fun, I think I'll stick around another year."

On December 29, 2000, Sister Esther Boor, the oldest living School Sister of Notre Dame, celebrated her 106th birthday.

Recommended Reading

A complete bibliography of Nun Study research publications, together with abstracts of the papers, is available on the Nun Study Web site: www.nunstudy.org.

Bell, Virginia and David Troxel. *The Best Friends Approach to Alzheimer's Care.* Baltimore: Health Professions Press, 1997.

Friel McGowin, Diana. *Living in the Labyrinth: A Personal Journey Through the Maze of Alzheimer's Disease.* New York: Delta Publishing, 1994.

Hayflick, Leonard. *How and Why We Age.* New York: Ballantine Books, 1996.

Johnson, Richard P. *The 12 Keys to Spiritual Vitality: Powerful Lessons on Living Agelessly.* Liguori, MO: Liguori, 1998.

Keck, David. *Forgetting Whose We Are: Alzheimer's Disease and the Love of God.* Nashville: Abingdon Press, 1996.

Kuhn, Daniel. *Alzheimer's Early Stages: First Steps in Caring and Treatment.* Alameda, CA: Hunter House, 1999.

Mace, Nancy L. and Peter V. Rabins. *The 36-Hour Day: A Family Guide to Caring for Persons with Alzheimer Disease, Related Dementing Illness and Memory Loss in Later Life.* Baltimore: Johns Hopkins University Press, 1999.

Perls, Thomas T., Margery Hutter Silver, and John F. Lauerman. *Living to 100: Lessons in Living to Your Maximum Potential at Any Age.* New York: Basic Books, 1999.

Rowe, John W., and Robert Louis Khan. *Successful Aging.* New York: Dell Publishing, 1999.

Tanzi, Rudolph E., and Ann B. Parson. *Decoding Darkness: The Search for the Genetic Causes of Alzheimer's Disease.* Cambridge, MA: Perseus Publishing, 2000.

Zgola, Jitka M. *Doing Things: A Guide to Programming Activities for Persons with Alzheimer's Disease and Related Disorders.* Baltimore: Johns Hopkins University Press, 1987.

OTHER SOURCES OF INFORMATION AND ASSISTANCE

Alzheimer's Association
919 North Michigan Avenue—Suite 1100
Chicago, IL 60611-1676
(800) 272-3900
(312) 335-8700
E-mail: info@alz.org
Web site: www.alz.org

Alzheimer's Disease Education and Referral Center
National Institute on Aging
P.O. Box 8250
Silver Spring, MD 20907-8250
(800) 438-4380
E-mail: adear@alzheimers.org
Web site: www.alzheimers.org

Alzheimer Research Forum
Web site: www.alzforum.org
Although this site is designed primarily to keep researchers
and physicians aware of the most recent developments in the
field, it includes valuable information for the general public.

Administration on Aging
330 Independence Avenue, SW
Washington, DC 20201
(800) 677-1116
E-mail: AoAInfo@aoa.gov
Web site: www.aoa.gov

American Association of Retired Persons (AARP)
601 E Street, NW
Washington, DC 20049
(800) 424-3410
E-mail: member@aarp.org
Web site: www.aarp.org

Information and referral services also can be obtained by con-
tacting your county office on aging, your local Area Agency on
Aging, or the U.S. Government's eldercare locator service at
(800) 677-1116.

Acknowledgments

This book would not have been possible without the spirited support of the members, archivists, research consultants, leaders, and health care providers of the School Sisters of Notre Dame congregation. In particular, I would like to recognize Sisters Gabriel Mary Spaeth, Marlene Manney, Rita Schwalbe, Mary Dominic Klaseus, Dolores Rauch, Nicolette Welter, Rosella Kreuzer, Suzanne René Sobczynski, Mary Ann Kuttner, Del Marie Rysavy, Mary Luke Baldwin, and Helen Reed.

The following colleagues were especially helpful and supportive: Sandra Perry Raybourne, Gari-Anne Patzwald, Jeanne Ray, James Mortimer, William Markesbery, Lydia Greiner, David Wekstein, Piero Antuono, Cecil Runyons, Kathleen Blomquist, Karen Cinnamond, Ann Tudor, Deborah Danner, Wallace Friesen, Dot Blair, Judith Evans, and Richard Suzman.

Leonard Schuman, Roland Phillips, and James Vaupel were instrumental in shaping my understanding of science and its power to improve people's lives.

Main funding for the Nun Study is provided by the National Institute on Aging, with other funding from the Kleberg Foundation and the Abercrombie Foundation.

I am also grateful to my agent, Gail Ross, for encouraging me to write this book. Howard Yoon helped me convey the warmth and humanity of the sisters; Jon Cohen helped me make the science accessible; and Toni Burbank, my editor at Bantam, artfully blended these elements.

Finally, I would like to thank my family and friends for all of their encouragement.

Index

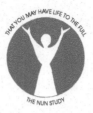

About the Nun Study

The Nun Study is an ongoing research program examining aging and Alzheimer's disease in a population of 678 U.S. members of the School Sisters of Notre Dame religious congregation. Dr. David Snowdon began this project as a pilot study in 1986. In 1990, funding by the National Institute on Aging permitted the study to expand into a large, multidisciplinary scientific and medical research project.

Participants in the Nun Study, who range in age from 75 to 106 years, allow investigators full access to their medical and convent records and undergo rigorous annual mental and physical testing. In addition, each participant has generously agreed to donate her brain at death. This wealth of historical and medical data has provided scientists with a unique view of aging and disease across the entire lifespan.

Research findings from the Nun Study have been published in prestigious scientific journals, including the *Journal of the American Medical Association* and the *Journal of Gerontology*, and have been reported in newspapers and magazines such as the *New York Times* and *National Geographic* as well as television programs such as *Nightline*. The Nun Study is one of several studies on aging and Alzheimer's disease being conducted at the Sanders-Brown Center on Aging, University of Kentucky Medical Center.

Further information about the Nun Study, including summaries of all research publications, is available on its Web site, www.nunstudy.org.

About the School Sisters of Notre Dame

The School Sisters of Notre Dame are members of an international congregation of Roman Catholic sisters. Originally founded in 1833 to teach poor girls, today's School Sisters of Notre Dame continue in the spirit of Christ, serving the poor and educating on all levels, with particular concern for youth and women. With a history rooted in service, they have missions in more than thirty countries in North America, Central America, South America, Europe, Africa, Asia, and Oceania.

Arriving in North America in 1847, they were among the early pioneers of Catholic education here, establishing thousands of schools throughout the United States. Today the School Sisters of Notre Dame incorporate their long-standing tradition as educators into all aspects of their service in diverse ministries, such as teaching, health and social services, justice and peace advocacy, spiritual direction, and parish and diocesan work.

Twenty-one provinces make up the worldwide network of School Sisters of Notre Dame, including seven in the United States. Although separated geographically, the School Sisters of Notre Dame are one in spirit, working together for the common good by empowering people to live fuller lives and to discover closer relationships with God.

School Sisters of Notre Dame
North American Major Area
www.ssnd.org

Baltimore Province
6401 North Charles Street
Baltimore, MD 21212-1099

Chicago Province
1431 Euclid Avenue
Berwyn, IL 60402-1216
www.ssndchicago.org

Dallas Province
4500 West Davis
P.O. Box 227275
Dallas, TX 75222-7275

Mankato Province
170 Good Counsel Drive
Mankato, MN 56001-3138
www.ssndmankato.org

Milwaukee Province
13105 Watertown Plank Road
Elm Grove, WI 53122-2291

St. Louis Province
320 East Ripa Avenue
St. Louis, MO 63125-2897

Wilton Province
345 Belden Hill Road
Wilton, CT 06897-3898

About the Author

David Snowdon was born and raised in southern California and received his Ph.D. in epidemiology in 1981 from the University of Minnesota. In 1990 he accepted a position at the University of Kentucky Medical Center. He is currently Professor of Neurology and Director of the Nun Study at the Sanders-Brown Center on Aging.

His ability to intertwine human stories with the excitement of scientific discovery has made him a popular speaker to both professional and lay audiences in the United States, Europe, and Africa.

Half of his proceeds from *Aging with Grace* will be donated to the School Sisters of Notre Dame.